R. D. Laing in the Twenty-First Century

In this remarkable review of the seminal contribution of the Scottish psychiatrist and psychoanalyst, R. D. Laing, the three authors, each intimately acquainted with the subject matter, explore Laing's intellectual and clinical legacy.

Written from the perspective of a psychoanalyst, a scientist, and a philosopher, this unique book thoroughly addresses the three principal themes that defined Laing's work: his views about sanity and madness, the use of therapy with those suffering from psychotic disturbance, and the vicissitudes of love relationships. They also explore authenticity, altered states, and healing. The authors bring a broad range of viewpoints in assessing Laing's seminal contribution to contemporary thought, from both a scholarly and personal assessment rooted in each of their diverse relationships with him, both professional and personal.

This volume will be of interest to those in the worlds of psychoanalysis, philosophy, science, and anyone with an interest in the work of R. D. Laing.

M. Guy Thompson, PhD, received his psychoanalytic training from R. D. Laing and colleagues at the Philadelphia Association in London and is the founder and director of the New School for Existential Psychoanalysis, a virtual certificate-based training program in existential psychoanalysis. He is the author of *The Legacy of R. D. Laing: An Appraisal of His Contemporary Relevance* [Ed.] (2015); *The Death of Desire: An Existential Study in Sanity and Madness* (2017; 2nd edition); and most recently, *Essays in Existential Psychoanalysis: On the Primacy of Authenticity* (2024), all published by Routledge. He lives in Berkeley, California.

Fritjof Capra, PhD, physicist and systems theorist, is the author of several international bestsellers, including *The Tao of Physics* and *The Web of Life*. He is the coauthor, with Pier Luigi Luisi, of the multidisciplinary textbook *The Systems View of Life*. Capra's online course (www.capracourse.net) is based on his textbook.

Douglas Kirsner, PhD, is Emeritus Professor of Philosophy and Psychoanalytic Studies at Deakin University, Melbourne. He is the author of *The Schizoid World of Jean-Paul Sartre* and *R. D. Laing and Unfree Associations: Inside Psychoanalytic Institutes*. His interest in Laing includes living in a Philadelphia Association household during the 1970s.

Philosophy & Psychoanalysis Book Series
Series Editor
Jon Mills

Philosophy & Psychoanalysis is dedicated to current developments and cutting-edge research in the philosophical sciences, phenomenology, hermeneutics, existentialism, logic, semiotics, cultural studies, social criticism, and the humanities that engage and enrich psychoanalytic thought through philosophical rigor. With the philosophical turn in psychoanalysis comes a new era of theoretical research that revisits past paradigms while invigorating new approaches to theoretical, historical, contemporary, and applied psychoanalysis. No subject or discipline is immune from psychoanalytic reflection within a philosophical context including psychology, sociology, anthropology, politics, the arts, religion, science, culture, physics, and the nature of morality. Philosophical approaches to psychoanalysis may stimulate new areas of knowledge that have conceptual and applied value beyond the consulting room reflective of greater society at large. In the spirit of pluralism, *Philosophy & Psychoanalysis* is open to any theoretical school in philosophy and psychoanalysis that offers novel, scholarly, and important insights in the way we come to understand our world.

Titles in this series:

For more information about this series, please visit: www.routledge.com/
Routledge-Handbooks-in-Religion/book-series

"How can there be a more relevant voice in our contemporary world than R. D. Laing? Is there anything to be more grateful for than sanity amidst this insanity, of healing amidst this suffering, of the altered states of psychosis amidst this lunacy, of love amidst this hatred? Laing was crucial to the founding of the human potential movement in the early 1960s. He is just as relevant today. Thompson, Capra, and Kirsner have brought us a series of essays, presented at **Esalen** over the past ten years, to remind us of this key legacy and why we should listen, intensely and carefully."

Jeffrey J. Kripal, *author of Esalen: America and*
the Religion of No Religion

"An authentic and scholarly work which greatly enriches the legacy of R. D. Laing's contribution to the experience-orientated philosophy of madness."

Adrian C. Laing, *Lawyer, author, son of R. D. Laing and*
author of R. D. Laing: A life *(Amazon Kindle),*
President: The R. D. Laing Estate: www.rdlaingofficial.com

"This fascinating book illuminates the influential work of the psychoanalyst and anti-psychiatrist R. D. Laing – a synthesizer of psychoanalysis with existentialist thought, Buddhism, family-systems theory, and cultural critique. Each essay in this volume was written by a thinker who knew Laing personally, knows his ideas intimately, and writes with clarity, sophistication, and verve. Laing was a crucial figure of the late 20th century. These erudite essays reveal his continuing relevance for our understanding of sanity and madness, of love and authenticity, of healing and altered states."

Louis Sass, *author of* Madness and Modernism *and*
The Paradoxes of Delusion.

"R. D. Laing in the 21st Century is essential reading for anyone concerned about the deeper levels of human freedom and community. The authors of this volume beautifully unpack Laing's "live and let live" philosophy for a new generation mystified by, and too often suffering from, ever widening forms of social coercion. While Thompson and his colleagues do not offer pat answers to this monumental plight, their Laing-inspired insights provide hope for a more loving, honesty-based world."

Kirk Schneider, *author of* The Psychology of Existence *(with Rollo May)*,
The Polarized Mind, *and* Life-Enhancing Anxiety: Key to a Sane World.

"The three authors, who knew and worked intimately with Laing, offer unique, illuminating understandings of his groundbreaking work. Importantly, they bring Laing into the 21st century to include our – hopefully not too late – ecological concerns of our interconnectedness, and such competing ideals as community and individual freedom. Through revisiting and contextually updating Laing's seminal writings, this stimulating and engaging book can help us come more to our senses with and through others, in our otherwise increasingly lonely and alienating world."

Del Loewenthal, *Emeritus Professor of Psychotherapy and Counselling, University of Roehampton, U.K., Chair of Existential Analytic Psychotherapy Training at the Southern Association for Psychotherapy and Counselling (SAFPAC) U.K., author of* Existential Psychotherapy and Counselling after Postmodernism *(Routledge, 2018). www.delloewenthal.com.*

R. D. Laing in the Twenty-First Century

Sanity, Therapy, Love

M. Guy Thompson, Fritjof Capra
and Douglas Kirsner

Routledge
Taylor & Francis Group

LONDON AND NEW YORK

Designed cover image: © John Haynes

First published 2025
by Routledge
4 Park Square, Milton Park, Abingdon, Oxon OX14 4RN

and by Routledge
605 Third Avenue, New York, NY 10158

Routledge is an imprint of the Taylor & Francis Group, an informa business

© 2025 M. Guy Thompson, Fritjof Capra and Douglas Kirsner

British Library Cataloguing-in-Publication Data
A catalogue record for this book is available from the British Library

ISBN: 978-1-032-91633-0 (hbk)
ISBN: 978-1-032-91632-3 (pbk)
ISBN: 978-1-003-56429-4 (ebk)

DOI: 10.4324/9781003564294

Typeset in Times New Roman
by Apex CoVantage, LLC

Contents

Preface

Themes From the Esalen Lectures

R. D. Laing wore many robes in his career, including psychiatrist, psychoanalyst, philosopher, social critic, author, poet, and mystic. At the peak of his fame and popularity in the 1970s he was the most widely read psychiatrist in the world. Renown of that magnitude is dependent on the happy coincidence of a multitude of factors, including the right message at the most opportune time. This was no doubt true for Laing, when the student unrest of the Vietnam War intersected with his devastating critique of a society, he argued, that was intent on subverting the minds of its youth for undisclosed purposes. At a time when authority figures of every persuasion were suspect, the counterculture embraced this hip, disarming Scotsman to explain how they were being mystified and why. Arguably the most controversial psychoanalyst since Freud, Laing's meteoric rise in the 1960s and 1970s was the result of his rare ability to make complex ideas accessible with such best-selling classics as *The Divided Self* (1960 [1969]); *Sanity, Madness and Family* (with Aaron Esterson, 1964 [1970]); *The Politics of Experience* (1967); *Knots* (1970); and many others. Laing's impassioned plea for a more humane treatment of those in society who are most vulnerable catapulted him into the vanguard of intellectual and cultural debate about the nature of sanity and madness and inspired a generation of psychology students, intellectuals, and artists to turn Laing into a cultural icon. His impact on the youth of the 1970s was especially pronounced in the United States, where his renown rivaled even that of the Indian gurus that were the rage among the college crowd's cognoscenti.

Laing's extraordinary reach into the American zeitgeist was based almost entirely on his devastating critique of conventional psychiatric practices, which he believed were often more sinister than the mental illness they presumed to treat. The (albeit reluctant) father of anti-psychiatry, Laing developed a daring alternative to conventional psychiatric treatment in 1965 at Kingsley Hall, the therapy center in London where he conceived the notion of a community where therapists and patients alike could live without clearly defined roles. This controversial treatment regimen was so successful that it continues to operate more than fifty years later and is even funded by the Local Council in London. Kingsley Hall also inspired numerous residential treatment communities in North America (Soteria House, Diabasis, Birch House, Shadows) that eventually led to a sea change in contemporary attitudes about the involuntary incarceration of the mentally ill.

But Laing not only innovated a unique approach to the residential treatment of the severely mentally ill. He also conceived a novel approach to psychoanalytic training, integrating Freud, Klein, and the Middle School with existential philosophy (Sartre, Heidegger, Nietzsche, Kierkegaard, Merleau-Ponty, and others) and Buddhism, especially the Zen and Chan traditions. (I founded Free Association, Inc., in 1988 in San Francisco, California, a not-for-profit 501©3 organization to further Laing's legacy, for the purpose of training a new generation of existential psychoanalysts in California, modeled on my training with Laing in London.)

Laing, who had studied philosophy as rigorously as he had the history and practice of psychiatry and psychoanalysis, sought to integrate existential philosophy and psychoanalysis after founding the Philadelphia Association in 1965. Much earlier, a group of European psychoanalytically trained psychiatrists, mostly German and French, in the post–World War II era of the 1940s and 1950s sought to integrate Martin Heidegger's existential philosophy into Freud's early conception of psychoanalysis – at that time, the only conception of psychoanalysis – with mixed results. Those psychoanalysts among us who were already schooled in existential philosophy and were trying our best to integrate it with Freudian psychoanalysis were thrilled with the publication of the American translations of many of these existential psychiatrists and analysts, titled *Existence* (1958), edited by Rollo May, and others appeared, introducing these writings into English for the first time. However, as interesting as these writings were, they were also virtually useless as an aid to learning how to practice a genuinely existential approach to psychoanalysis. After a decade or two of avid interest among American therapists who had been schooled or were just interested in existential philosophy and appearing in American journals devoted to existential psychology, the movement petered out around the time Laing's notoriety peaked. It was Laing's renown in the early 1970s that inspired me to abandon my doctoral studies in San Francisco to study with Laing in 1973.

Of course, it was Laing's books that made him world famous, many of which continue to sell at an impressive rate. *The Divided Self*; *Sanity, Madness and the Family*; *The Politics of Experience*; and *Knots* are now considered classics and continue to serve as the foundation of Laing's unique and disconcerting message. They are just as relevant today, and just as radical, as when they were first published in the 1960s and 1970s.

On a broader cultural level Laing's ideas spread far beyond matters concerning psychotherapy and the treatment of the mentally ill. Nearly every American college student in the early 1970s was reading *The Politics of Experience*, a campus bestseller that seemed to encapsulate the undercurrent of social malaise that so many young people were then feeling. When the pot-smoking, acid-dropping counterculture intersected with the radical anti–Vietnam War protest movement, Laing's critique of how people in power were systematically mystifying them transformed him into a social phenomenon and quasi-spiritual leader. So what was his message and why was its impact so palpable?

Laing died in 1989 at the age of 62. As we were approaching the 25th anniversary of Laing's death in 2013, I decided to organize a symposium in New York City to honor Laing's legacy. I invited a number of therapists, academics, and thinkers who had all known Laing personally, either in the UK or the United States, to convene for a weekend at Wagner College on Staten Island to share lectures on Laing's enduring impact on contemporary culture. Fritjof Capra and Douglas Kirsner, the other two contributors to this volume, were featured speakers among many others. The papers presented there were subsequently published by Routledge under the title, *The Legacy of R. D. Laing: An Appraisal of His Contemporary Relevance* (2015). The book you are now reading effectively serves as a sequel to that publication.

After the intense interest that followed this highly successful symposium, I decided to host more symposia devoted to Laing's legacy, but on an annual basis, and to move the venue for these meetings from New York to California, at the renowned Esalen Institute in Big Sur. Esalen's relationship with Laing is of historic importance due to Laing's frequent visits there, beginning in the mid-1960s and culminating toward the end of the 1980s with Laing's death. In 1968, Richard Price and Michael Murphy, two Stanford dropout psychologists who were profoundly unhappy with conventional psychiatry, convened a summer-long series of symposia under the title, "The Value of Psychotic Experience" at Esalen, a retreat center on the Pacific Ocean owned by the Murphy family. These meetings were designed to explore the meaning of sanity and madness, altered states of consciousness, and humane alternatives to conventional psychiatric treatment for those suffering from extreme states. Participants in addition to Laing included Aldous Huxley, Gregory Bateson, Abraham Maslow, Fritz Perls, John Perry, Stan Grof, Julian Silverman, Alan Watts, and others. All participants shared their respective experiences and thoughts about psychotic states and altered states of consciousness.

It was on this occasion that Laing first shared his groundbreaking work at Kingsley Hall in London (founded in 1965). Laing's experiences at Kingsley Hall helped inspire Julian Silverman to initiate the Agnews Project in San Jose, out of which evolved Loren Mosher's residential treatment center at Soteria House, loosely modeled on Kingsley Hall. A few years later two San Francisco Jungian analysts, John Perry and Howard Levine, initiated a similar project, Diabasis, in San Francisco. Esalen's role in bringing all of these extraordinary thinkers together for the first time was instrumental in creating opportunities for alternative treatment modalities to flourish all over America. What all of these projects shared in common was seeking alternative ways of understanding extreme forms of consciousness that were opposed to the medicalization of madness, so-called "mental illness." This was essential to Laing's perspective and carried over in the Soteria and Diabasis projects. Neither of these projects necessarily saw themselves as "treating mental illness," but rather in helping people who had lost their way come to their senses, in time, but with little or no conventional "treatment" of any kind.

A considerable amount of time has passed since the experimental 1960s and 1970s, but Esalen continues to host workshops and symposia that are now identified with the human potential movement. Though Richard Price passed away decades ago, Michael Murphy lives on (he is in his 90s) and continues to host his research-oriented Center for Theory and Research (CTR), also housed at Esalen. Despite Esalen's current focus on workshops devoted to yoga, dance, spirituality, and the like, I envisioned Esalen as the perfect home for furthering Laing's legacy due to its history of innovating new forms of therapy, including gestalt, encounter groups, and symposia on psychosis and alternative modes of healing.

With this brief history, I now want to turn our attention to the lectures contained in this volume, all of which were given by the authors of this collection of essays. All of them occurred at our annual Esalen Symposia between 2015 and 2023. The purpose of the annual R. D. Laing in the Twenty-First Century symposia was to bring a taste of what it was like to study and train with Laing at his Philadelphia Association in London and to keep alive his legacy as an icon for alternatives to conventional psychiatry. What was most remarkable about participating in Laing's study center was the uncommon informality and Laing's explicitly non-academic approach to exploring the most fundamental aspects of the human condition. In the spirit of Martin Heidegger, Laing brought to bear in his teaching a manner of questioning – and questing – into topics as fundamental as sanity and madness, authenticity, healing, love, altered states, and so on. These meetings were personal in the extreme, and though the thinkers under study were the most important philosophers in the Western canon, you wouldn't get what Laing and his cohorts were saying about them and how relevant they are to healing at any university!

Similarly, at our Esalen symposia we wanted to provide a forum where such ideas could be explored openly and openheartedly, not pedantically. The emphasis was on discussing ideas with everyone present, on an equal basis. These were not messages from "on high." Our intention was not to pretend that we had all the answers to the questions we posed. The most essential questions about the human condition offer no easy or universal answers. As you will see, even the title of the themes we selected for each symposium are posed as questions.

The symposia were originally organized by myself (M. Guy Thompson), Nita Gage (who also trained as a therapist with Laing), and Fritjof Capra (who engaged with Laing in many inspiring and challenging discussions during the last ten years of Laing's life).

We decided that each year the three of us would select a theme that we believed was close to Laing's heart and about which guided much of Laing's thinking, sourced from publications, non-published materials, and personal conversations with Laing. Though there are usually a dozen speakers or so who participate at each of our symposia, the three of us were assigned the task of explicitly exploring Laing's ideas and articulating them as accessibly as possible. We did not have the space to include every single paper we gave at each symposium in this volume, so what you see here, outlined in the Table of Contents, is a selection of the symposia we believe are most representative of what we were able to accomplish.

I will now go over the themes we decided to include and the papers that each of us presented.

In our inaugural Esalen symposium in July 2015 the theme of our meeting was What Is Sanity? What Is Madness? Our aim was to explore the most seminal question at the heart of nearly every book Laing published, including *The Divided Self*; *Self and Others*; *Sanity, Madness and the Family*; *The Politics of Experience*; *Knots*; *The Politics of the Family*; and so on. In Chapter 1, I explore the healing element of Portland Road, the post–Kingsley Hall residential healing residence that I lived in for four years in the 1970s. In Chapter 2, Douglas Kirsner reviews the gist of Laing's views on sanity and madness from both published and unpublished books and lectures given by Laing. In Chapter 3, Fritjof Capra explores contemporary examples of everyday madness that often go unnoticed because they are so common. (Everyday madness was a favorite theme of Laing's.)

In 2016, the theme of our symposium was What Is Therapeutic? In Chapter 4, I chose to explore the nature of sympathy and its relation to empathy in the therapeutic process, a favorite theme of Laing's that was inspired by his reading of Max Scheler's philosophical work, *The Nature of Sympathy* (1954). Next, In Chapter 5, Douglas Kirsner explores Laing's surprisingly scant publications as well as unpublished lectures on this topic. And finally, in Chapter 6, Fritjof Capra chose to explore the relation between science and spirituality, focusing on the therapeutic element of spirituality.

In 2017, the theme of our symposium was What Are Altered States? Though this term is often associated with psychedelic drugs, such as LSD, we wanted to address the concept in its widest application, including mindfulness, meditation, yoga, extraordinary feeling states, and the like. In Chapter 7, Fritjof Capra explores the concept of reality in its scientific, spiritual, and philosophical aspects. In Chapter 8, I chose to explore how falling in love manifests a very special example of altered states, in this case initiated by emotions. In Chapter 9, Douglas Kirsner explored Laing's use of LSD in a therapeutic context at Kingsley Hall, drawing on an unpublished lecture that Laing gave at the William Alanson White Institute in New York.

In 2018, we turned our attention to the seminal question, What Is Love?, a critical theme in all of Laing's writings. In Chapter 10, I chose to explore the relation between eros and agapé, the erotic and spiritual dimensions of love, initiated by the Greeks (Eros and Agapé were deities in Greek folklore). Whereas eros comes to us primarily from Plato's dialogue, *The Symposium*, and influenced both Sigmund Freud's and Laing's respective applications of erotic love to their understanding of madness, agapé became a central element in Christianity, in both Catholic and Protestant editions. Next, in Chapter 11, Fritjof Capra focuses on the biology of love, grounded in life's pervasive tendency to interconnect and interrelate. Finally, in Chapter 12, Douglas Kirsner reviews Laing's many references to love in both his published work and unpublished lectures.

In 2019, our theme was What Is Authenticity? Next to sanity and madness, there is likely no other theme closer to Laing's heart than the explicitly existential and philosophical exploration of the importance of honesty in our human relationships, both in our relations with others and with ourselves. In Chapter 13, Douglas Kirsner reviews Laing's many references to the concept of authenticity in both published work and unpublished lectures, manifested primarily in Laing's notion of true and false self-phenomena, a preoccupation Laing shared with D. W. Winnicott, the renowned British psychoanalyst who was also Laing's supervisor in his psychoanalytic training in London. In Chapter 14, I chose to explore the dark side of Laing's personal relationship with authenticity, supposedly due to the controversial nature of Laing's way of seizing on every opportunity in his relationships with friends, students, and confidants to demonstrate aspects of how authenticity shows up in everyday life; not always to their pleasure! Finally, in Chapter 15, Fritjof Capra explores the relationship between authenticity and community, drawing heavily from Capra's many publications on a new systemic understanding of life which has emerged at the forefront of science over the past 30 years.

Skipping ahead to 2023, the theme of our annual symposium that year was What Is Healing? We believed it was fitting to open our selection of themes in this volume with exploring sanity and madness and to close with what is entailed in healing. I open with an exploration of the etymology of the word "heal," which is cognate with the word "sane," or sanity, and argue that healing and sanity come from similar roots but in a non-medicalized context. Next, in Chapter 17, Fritjof Capra explores the concept of a "systems view of health," examining in particular the relation between health and regeneration, a principal aspect of maintaining healthy living. And finally, in Chapter 18, our final chapter, Douglas Kirsner explores Laing's thoughts about the human condition, drawing primarily on a seminal interview that Kirsner conducted with Laing in 1980, as well as Laing's crucial relationship with the philosophy of Jean-Paul Sartre, perhaps the most famous of all the existential philosophers.

What all these lectures have in common is that they were written by three thinkers who knew Laing personally and who were profoundly influenced by both his person and his ideas. In this, these lectures and the book they contain are unique. They are based on the premise that only those who knew Laing, both personally and professionally, truly understood him and his unique meditation on the human condition. We hope that you will enjoy reading them as much as we have enjoyed sharing our explorations of Laing's legacy over the past ten years. It has been a work of love for all of us, and we sincerely hope that this decade of devoting ourselves to the question who was R. D. Laing will bear fruit.

M. Guy Thompson, PhD

References

Laing, R. D. (1960[1969]). *The divided self: An existential study in sanity and madness.* New York and London: Penguin Books.

Laing, R. D. (1967). *The politics of experience.* New York: Ballentine Books.

Laing, R. D. and Esterson, A. (1964[1970]). *Sanity, madness and the family*. New York and London: Penguin Books.

May, R., Angel, E., and Ellenberger, H. (Eds.) (1958). *Existence: A new dimension in psychiatry and psychology* (Various Trans.). New York: Basic Books.

Scheler, M. (1954). *The nature of sympathy* (Peter Heath, Trans.). London: Routledge and Kegan Paul.

Thompson, M. Guy (ed.) (2015). *The legacy of R. D. Laing: An appraisal of his contemporary relevance*. London and New York: Routledge.

1

What Is Sanity? What Is Madness?

Chapter 1

Sanity and Friendship
The Therapeutic Feature of Communal Living

M. Guy Thompson, PhD

In the early 1970s I became acquainted with the work of R. D. Laing, and in 1973 I decided to relocate from California to London to work with him. I thought I would stay there a year and then return to my graduate studies in San Francisco. Instead I stayed for seven years, seven remarkable years that changed my life. During that time I trained as a psychoanalyst, and for four of those years I lived in one of Laing's post–Kingsley Hall communities, Portland Road. While there, I met my future wife, and our two sons were born in London before we eventually returned to the United States.

Laing had become internationally famous for his radical experiment with alternative ways of treating schizophrenia. In fact, in 1973, the year I went to work with him, Laing was the most famous psychiatrist in the world. He was brilliant and charismatic and the prolific author of numerous best-selling works, including *The Divided Self* (1960[1969]) and *The Politics of Experience* (1967). In 1965 Laing established Kingsley Hall, a residential household for people who wanted an alternative to mental hospitals. There were no paid staff, and no one had an assigned role, yet many therapists also lived there, including Laing. It was, as he put it, a "melting pot where preconceptions were melted down in the nitty-gritty of living together." Laing obviously had a way with words!

As no formal treatment was provided for the residents living there, many of whom had been diagnosed as schizophrenic when previously in hospital, the question I want to pose here is: What was the healing or therapeutic agent of living in such a community if no ostensible treatment was provided? If we decide to abandon psychiatric nomenclature and the very concept of "treatment," even group therapy, then how can healing ostensibly occur? My talk will make reference to both Kingsley Hall and Portland Road – Kingsley Hall because that is where Laing conceived this model, and Portland Road because that is the community I was involved with and the one that I believe perfected this approach.

Part I

Both Kingsley Hall and Portland Road were informed by Laing's depiction of the schizoid personality, as illustrated in *The Divided Self* as a distinctive form of

DOI: 10.4324/9781003564294-2

alienation that these residential household communities were best suited for relieving. Laing believed that the schizoid person is alienated in a double sense. Because the schizoid individual is suffering from catastrophic anxiety, what Laing termed *ontological insecurity*, such a person is profoundly averse to getting too close to others, for fear that others will "engulf" him by compromising what is left of his fragile autonomy. On the other hand, this person is just as anxious about being utterly alone in the world, isolated and estranged from others. So he threads a needle, as it were, between engulfment on the one extreme and isolation on the other, until the piece of ground he is clinging to is little more than the edge of a precipice. This is a very precarious place to be, not knowing whom to turn to or where to go to be safe. Laing conceived Kingsley Hall as a refuge or sanctuary where you would be protected from being engulfed by others but surrounded by compassionate people, many of whom are more or less like yourself. The premium there was on *asylum*, a safe place to be where you could have a room of your own if you wanted, where you could stay for as long as you wished.

By the time I arrived in London in 1973, Kingsley Hall had closed and was replaced by two household communities, the Archway Community and Portland Road, named after the neighborhoods in London, where they were located. I opted to live in Portland Road and went into therapy with the psychoanalyst who established that household, Hugh Crawford. At this stage Laing was no longer involved with the houses directly.

Hugh Crawford was profoundly influenced by Laing's depiction of the pre-schizophrenic, schizoid personality, who on the outer edge of a diagnostic continuum is usually diagnosed as schizophrenic. Crawford also agreed that the principal dilemma facing the typical resident at Portland Road was the feeling of alienation, from others as well as from oneself. To live in a state of alienation is to be without love. It is a loveless existence, and that is the crux of the issue. Without love, life has no meaning or purpose. It is an empty and heartless place to be and a form of existence that is fundamentally intolerable.[1] Consequently, Crawford saw that person's redemption differently than Laing did. For Crawford, relief from chronic isolation was the more pressing issue, so no one was guaranteed a room of one's own at Portland Road. Everyone shared. Like Buddhist monasteries, privacy was neither a premium nor a virtue. What was emphasized was *togetherness*. Crawford believed that such people were already experts at living incognito, whether in the company of others or by themselves, so why encourage them with more of the same? The challenge was to generate an ambience of conviviality that would not feel threatening, but inviting. If people who came to live at Portland Road typically found relationships intrusive and artificial, then efforts should be made to offer ways of engaging with them that were protective, but *real*. Laing's and Crawford's respective views represented two very different interpretations of how to address this problem, from two very different personalities. Common wisdom at the Philadelphia Association was that Laing was the head of the organization but that Crawford was its heart. For those of you familiar with the history of psychoanalysis, Crawford was Ferenczi to Laing's Freud.

Another way of articulating this distinction is that Portland Road was based on the healing power of facilitating relationships with others in the form of a special type of friendship. This was rooted in Crawford's observation that the schizophrenic is a person "who has no friends" and needs opportunities to make friends with people he or she would otherwise avoid. So what kind of friendship are we talking about among people who have never been inclined to risk friendship before?

Aristotle on Friendship

Aristotle talks about three distinct kinds of friendship: the fair-weather friend, the collegial friend, and the true or genuine friend. Only true friendship endures, because it's the only type of friendship that is predicated on accepting each other for who each person is and loving that person accordingly. Residents at Portland Road craved this kind of friendship but were also afraid of it. By living together without any treatment program or overt therapy taking place, even group therapy, people were free to form meaningful relationships with each other so that, in time, they eventually formed alliances with one or more of the people living there. This process occurred haphazardly and spontaneously, with no overt efforts at matchmaking. To do so would have felt contrived.

Now I want to make a few observations about the nature of friendship and how this pertains to communities such as Portland Road. Aristotle (2011, p. 181) once remarked: "Friendship seems to be the bond that holds communities together." The Greek word for friendship was *philia*, one of the three prevalent Greek words for love, with *eros* and *agapé* being the other two. Laing named his organization the Philadelphia Association, which derives from the word, *philia*, because he conceived it as a brotherhood or sisterhood of friends. This means that friendship is a form of love, and without love as the essential element, you have no friendship. *Philia*, as I am guessing you know, is also the root for the word "philosophy," which literally means a love – or *friend* – of wisdom.

So what about these three forms of friendship that Aristotle talked about? Each one is rooted in the pursuit of the things in life that we love the most. The most basic is the love of pleasure, embodied in friendships with whom we share valued activities and interests. The second is characterized by our love of work, so this would include people with whom we conduct commerce, earn our living, and the relationships that help us survive. The third is the most mysterious kind of friendship and arguably the most rare. Aristotle refers to this as simply the "true" or genuine friend. This is the most intimate kind of friendship because it is the friend I'm willing to share everything with, who I hide nothing from. This is the kind of friend I can count on when the chips are down. This is also a friend who I would never judge and who would never judge me, who accepts me for who I am. This is the kind of friend I would die for.

It's this third kind of friendship that Hugh Crawford was hoping to nurture at Portland Road. What I find most interesting about this form of friendship is its power to *transform*. Freud conceived the analytic relationship as one in which the therapist never passes judgment on the patient, embodied in his concept of neutrality. He believed that this lack of judgment is so unexpected that when we encounter it in the context of a therapeutic relationship, it elicits a potentially transformative experience. We experience a sense of intimacy that is so powerful, we nearly always feel a special affection for our therapist.

But the most important thing to take home about these three types of friendship is that, ideally, we find elements of each in every friend who we love. Every friendship has the potential for shared joy, for making us more productive, and for feeling better about ourselves, as a consequence of the acceptance we derive from each other. This is the kind of friendship that is the bedrock of successful marriages. The British psychoanalyst Masud Khan added a fourth type of friendship that he characterized as "crucial" friendship, modeled on the therapy experience. This is a friendship that is so accepting of who you are as a person that it has the power to open your heart and to make you into a more loving person. I prefer to call this a *mutative* friendship, due to its power to transform. This is ideally the kind of friendship you enjoyed with your own therapist, if you were very lucky.

Let Me Summarize What I've Said So Far

- A friend is someone in whose company we take pleasure.
- Friendships are *enduring*. You may have a one-off sexual encounter with a seductive stranger you'll never see again, but a friend is a person you *want* to see again, and again, and again.
- As noted earlier, Aristotle believed that friendships form a bond that holds a community together. But not all communities are bound by friendship. Most communities are composed of people who don't necessarily take delight in being together, who may enjoy some degree of conviviality or companionship, but who basically put up with each other. They may dutifully, even earnestly, try as they may, contractually help each other. But such communities, strictly speaking, are not founded on *friendship*, because the people involved don't love each other.
- For Aristotle, even friendships that are rooted exclusively in the pursuit of pleasure, such as friends who share a passion for golf or the movies, are nevertheless cemented by a shared interest that bonds them together, in common cause, through which they experience mutual delight – even when these activities are the sole basis of the friendship.
- Another ingredient of friendship is the mutual dependency and trust shared between friends, especially when one of them gets into trouble. This quality of mutual reliance is an essential element to all friendships, for without trust and mutual regard, you can't really love the other person.
- Not all commercial relationships are rooted in love. Business relations where people merely use one another for personal gain or advantage, with a disregard for the other's welfare, don't offer the ingredients for what Aristotle characterizes as a friendship rooted in *philia*. The business acquaintance who, after he's

cut your throat, says that you shouldn't "take it personally," that "it's only business," is not much of a friend.

- Groups and institutions in which *philia* is absent are the norm in mental hospitals. On a more subtle level, *philia* is absent even in most groups that aspire to become therapeutic communities, that may champion what they depict as social, or community, even a milieu approach to "group therapy." Instead, they compensate for the absence of *philia* with modes of communication that are technological in nature.

They feed on contrived and incessant "feedback," a technique for forcibly baring your feelings, whether you want to share those feelings or not, in the guise of "check-ins" and other convoluted modes of pseudo-communication. Here, technology has replaced the more simple, if elusive, opportunity for developing genuine friendship. I'm not talking about the technology of medication, or straitjackets, or lobotomy, but the calculated use of conversation that passes for getting to know one another.

Ideally, friendships have a crucial bearing on what people living in therapeutic communities get from the experience and whether they can say that the time living there was genuinely worthwhile. It goes without saying that life in any community that conceives of itself as therapeutic, including those that dispense with therapeutic interventions, isn't going to be easy.

What I'm characterizing as fostering meaningful, intimate friendships in communal settings is the consequence of two essential factors.

- Such communities are focused on helping people who've never learned how to form intimate relations with others, who've historically found relationships more painful than rewarding. These communities don't try to develop "self-sufficiency," but rather *mutual dependency* as a catalyst for developing genuine fellowship with others.
- The therapeutic element in these places is subtle. It is rooted in nothing more complex than the attentiveness that each participant is encouraged to direct on *oneself in relation to everyone else* in the community. You might call this kind of attentiveness a form of meditation, because by it we focus our attention on the life that we're sharing with others, in the day-to-day, nitty-gritty excitement and boredom that comprises any domestic relationship.

This is a necessarily arduous discipline. Because of its inherently unpredictable nature, periods of dissatisfaction and malaise are inevitable. In fact, such incidents of disenchantment and anguish are valuable. The aim isn't to achieve a semblance of contrived cheerfulness that is mandated, for example, in summer camp or on cruise ships. Instead, the aim, as in psychotherapy, is to make a space for each person's suffering and allow that suffering to breathe, unmolested. This way we learn to respect each other's pain when it arises and embrace it, even when we are affected by it.

This is because the feeling that I am accepted by others, no matter how miserable or difficult I am to live with, elicits a sense of freedom that is itself healing.

I've noted three facets of friendship that have a bearing on the atmosphere that people living together may share: the enjoyment we feel in the company of others, the regard we invariably experience for a person we love, and the encouragement we derive from being part of a community that we genuinely belong to. My thesis is that friendships are not only desirable but an essential precondition for the well-being of any community, especially one that aspires to be therapeutic.

Part II

Now I want to turn my attention to the problem of isolation and alienation that is so characteristic of people who live in these places. According to Heidegger, the experience of loneliness, isolation, and alienation and their accompanying sense of homelessness are not limited to the schizoid or schizophrenic individuals described by Laing in *The Divided Self*. Heidegger believed that these characteristics are not solely symptomatic of people suffering from "psychopathology," but essential aspects of the human condition we all share. These so-called symptoms aren't, strictly speaking, pathological, but existential. Some experience these bouts of loneliness and alienation more profoundly than others, but none of us are strangers to what it feels like to be lonely and afraid.

People who get diagnosed as suffering from a psychotic something or other are at the extremities of what our culture, any culture, is prepared to tolerate. There is little sympathy for people who remind us of the private fears we hold inside and conceal from others. There's no way of connecting with such people without accessing that part of our own selves that is intimately familiar with what those fears are like. The reason that friendship and community are important to those so alienated is because intimacy makes us whole again by providing a sense of belonging to something and someone bigger than ourselves.

It is the experience of being a part of something bigger than me that is the basis of the spiritual experience, the feeling of being loved by the world I live in.

One of the pastimes that friends value the most is the time they spend together simply *conversing*. When we engage in conversation with a friend who is dear to us, we treasure the opportunity to share the things that concern us, including the things we like to complain about. This is why Freud made conversation his so-called treatment regimen. We crave conversation with others because it is the source of how we experience intimacy, by disclosing who we are to someone we trust will value our point of view. Toward the end of his life Freud concluded that talking to each other in this way is so powerful that he labeled his method the "talking cure."

There seems to be a continuum along a scale whereby the healthier a person is, the easier it becomes to self-disclose in this way. This is why the so-called schizophrenic finds this kind of disclosure so frightening. Dare he or she risk being that vulnerable and transparent to others?

So, how did the pursuit of friendship manifest at Portland Road, and what types of friendships resulted? For one thing, I'd have to admit that the kinds of friendships I've been describing were not typical there. If anything, the friendships formed at Portland Road were paradoxical and often one-sided. The pursuit of pleasure was rarely apparent. We're talking about people who, for the most part, had no previous experience of friendship. You might say that most of the people living there regarded each other in the same way that porcupines make love: *cautiously!* Those of us who weren't as crazy formed friendships readily with each other, but what about those who were paranoid or schizophrenic or unremittingly depressed?

Portland Road was a complicated yet carefully orchestrated mix of individuals with varied motives for being there. At its peak, fourteen people shared the house, which contained seven bedrooms. The people were more or less divided into two groups, sometimes not that distinct from each other. The larger group comprised people who had either spent some time in a mental hospital or would have had they not found their way to Portland Road. The other group comprised people, like myself, who had no history of a psychotic break but who lived there because we wanted to experience what it would be like, or because we wanted to be a part of Laing's mission to change the world, or because we were struggling with problems of our own that we believed living in such an environment would prove helpful for us. We may have been in the Philadelphia Association's analytic training program and wanted to deepen our understanding of sanity and madness. Or we may have been in therapy with Hugh Crawford, and he may have persuaded us to give it a try. The motives could be many and complex, and no doubt most of them were unconscious.

Whatever our motives may have been, it was crucial to the success of Portland Road that relatively healthy or sane people wanted to be a part of it. Without them, who would take it upon themselves to buy groceries, do the cooking and cleaning, and add an element of enjoyment to the experience? Without such people the place would have been depressing. This core group easily made friends with one another and were bound together in a way that reminded me of my experience in Vietnam, a kind of esprit de corp. It was those of us who were able to form friendships who were the first to befriend the other, more insulated residents of the house. So what were friendships like for them, and how successful were they in fostering their own friendships?

Because of the degree of estrangement that many of the people living at Portland Road endured, whatever friendships they formed with each other had something of a quality of "shared insularity," a state, you might say, of *friend-lessness.* Due to the emphasis on authentically being who you are, a kind of celebration of being different also contributed to the absence of friendly overtures. A degree of friendship was sometimes broached in an ironic sense, when two people backing in retreat from the outside world kind of "bump into" each other. They might like one another to a degree, but if a genuine friendship is to flourish, there has to be an overt turning about and *facing* each other. This requires a change of heart from the ordinary resentful, insolent attitude toward the world that characterized the typical resident living there. It's hard to make friends when you resent the life that you're living, when you have had little success at finding happiness.

While people at Portland Road were perfectly free to make friends, they were also free to *not* make friends. Fear of compliance and behaving the way "one is expected to" may serve as a powerful motive to deliberately not be friendly to others, for the sake of a sad attempt at behaving authentically. Most of the people living there were in open rebellion against the dictates of conventional society and the public false self that the healthy person accepts as a matter of course but that for the paranoid schizophrenic is perceived as an abdication of control and personal integrity. From this position, it may be difficult to comprehend the virtue of friendship. After all, it may be to them a kind of Trojan horse designed to get inside one's psyche for ulterior motives.

Yet this was only one side of the equation. The residents were not only wary of the potential dangers of intimacy. They also had problems with being on their own, with a limited capacity to enjoy their own company or to pursue their own interests. Consequently, they tended to find their self-imposed solitude unbearable. It was in this context that risks were sometimes taken, when they might share a moment of conviviality with another person. Because they were able to witness the kinds of friendships forming among the more social members of the community, they also had an opportunity to get a sense of how eagerly some people wanted to be intimate with others. For some, given the families they came from, this may have been the first time they ever witnessed people treating each other with genuine affection, and even love.

Because of their deeply ingrained distrust of others, Hugh Crawford dispensed with conventional "group therapy." One of the deadliest instruments of torture that I witnessed in mental hospitals was the group therapy sessions that all the patients were required to attend. Even I felt acutely uncomfortable in these settings, and I was a student with a badge of invulnerability. Yet I could easily recognize the subtle efforts to persuade patients to share their deepest feelings with everyone on command and to respond appropriately to the staff's efforts to get them out of their shell and to "be nice."

Portland Road dispensed with coercive efforts of this nature. Instead, we shared dinner together, then gathered in the kitchen or living room for post-dinner conversation. Usually, one person would ask Hugh Crawford something or other and begin to converse with him. Similar to Fritz Perls's conception of gestalt therapy but without the "hot seat," Crawford would share a conversation with this person while the rest of us listened on, enraptured. The focus for the evening would be on that person and that person alone, lost in conversation, with the rest of us keenly attentive to what this person was disclosing to us. It was clear to me that this was Crawford's way of forming friendships with each of the people living there.

Many of us were in individual therapy with Crawford, but it wasn't required or expected. The more regressed members of the community were typically loathe to leave the house, so the visits by Crawford were opportunities they seized on to connect with him, sometimes in desperation. Somehow this worked. I'm not sure how, but without Crawford's presence and obvious love that he had for everyone living there, I don't think it could have worked. It was this experience that finally brought home to me Freud's admonition that psychoanalysis is a cure through love.

It is difficult, perhaps impossible, to comprehend how a therapeutic community such as Kingsley Hall or Portland Road can be therapeutic with no ostensible therapy. This, I think, was an aspect of both Laing's and Crawford's genius. To recognize that what we typically conceive of as therapy is simply too contrived to help most people, especially those who are wary of contrivances of any kind. Instead, they believed that households of this nature could only work if, in lieu of this or that treatment regimen, you bring people together for no other purpose than to live together, like people all over the world manage to do, as naturally and intimately as possible. This can only be done, as Laing once noted, in the spirit of live and let live. As in any relationship, when the chips are down, you take your chances and I'll take mine, in the to and fro, wear and tear, of sharing my life with the community I am a part of, for better or for worse.

Note

1 See my book, *The Death of Desire: An Existential Study in Sanity and Madness* (2016), Chapter 7, for a more thorough exploration of the relation between love and madness.

References

Aristotle (2011). *Aristotle's Nichomachean ethics* (Robert Bartlett and Susan Collins, Trans.). Chicago and London: The University of Chicago Press.

Laing, R. D. (1960[1969]). *The divided self: An existential study in sanity and madness.* New York and London: Penguin Books.

Laing, R. D. (1967). *The politics of experience.* New York: Ballantine Books.

Thompson, M. Guy (2016). *The death of desire: An existential study in sanity and madness.* New York and London: Routledge.

Chapter 2

Laing on Sanity, Liberty, and Freedom

Douglas Kirsner, PhD

Individual agency and freedom underpin Laing's approach to sanity and madness. In this chapter, I want to explore these ideas within a context of the history of ideas, and I will stress Laing's strong belief in the value of individual freedom. Not only does this concern existential-phenomenological freedom but significantly involves political freedom in the liberal democratic tradition, resonating in particular with the British philosopher John Stuart Mill's classic 1859 essay *On Liberty* (Mill, 1859[2002]).

There Mill stresses the intrinsic value of individual political freedom and sees the inherent dangers of the tyranny of the majority. This goes beyond the results-driven utilitarianism that Mill also advocates – the greatest happiness for the greatest number. For Mill, the state has no right to intervene in people's lives and coerce them for their own good if they are not harming others. (Also related is how high the bar is for 'harm' to others – Mill's view was that harm meant way more than offence or hurt feelings that have come to be part of our contemporary politically correct culture.) For Laing, doing things to the patient 'for their own good' goes against the value of individual freedom.

But why is individual freedom such a central value? There are both principled and utilitarian reasons. On utilitarian grounds alone, it is all too easy to harm others; what is 'for your own good' is difficult, if not impossible, to decide, as things so easily go wrong. The voice of the patient may not be factored into an increasingly technocratic calculus.

According to Laing, sanity and madness involve a radical disjunction – a disjunction between a person who by common consent is sane and one whom common consent ascribes that radical difference. As Laing asserts in *The Divided Self*,

> The kernel of the schizophrenic's experience of himself must remain incomprehensible to us. As long as we are sane and he is insane, it will remain so . . . we have to recognize all the time his distinctiveness and differentness, his separateness and loneliness and despair.
>
> (Laing, 1960/1965, p. 38)

What kind of difference? In his psychiatric classic, *General Psychopathology*, Karl Jaspers declares that an 'abyss of difference' characterizes the relationship

DOI: 10.4324/9781003564294-3

between a sane person, exemplified by a psychiatrist, and a psychotic. Jaspers asserts that there is an unbridgeable gap between them and that such patients are 'un-understandable' (see Kirsner, 1990). Or as Eugen Bleuler, the Swiss psychiatrist who invented the term 'schizophrenia' in 1908, puts it, schizophrenics were stranger to him than the birds in his garden (Laing, 1965 p. 28). The idea of an unbridgeable gulf between sane and insane is alien to Laing's sensibility that always questions the distinction between us and them. I suspect this was rooted in the fact that, as it happened, Laing was able to hear and potentially understand a peculiarly broad range of experience.

Laing's starting point is that psychotics and sane people live along a continuum. The difference is not of kind, but of degree. Laing assumes that all humans are agents who choose their actions in some way or other. His existential approach means that we understand or decipher the experience and meaning in the actions of a psychotic instead of viewing the actions as mechanisms. Thus, for Laing, whatever their sanity, the behaviour of human beings is not the result of mechanisms or impulses, but, more than is normally assumed, emanates from choices.

Moreover, human beings are almost always in relationship, and these relationships have considerable impact upon perceptions and self-perceptions. Communications through language should be interpreted as potentially intentional, even where the communications appear to be meaningless. Such meaning relates not just to an inner world but also to family relationships and communications. As Laing suggests,

> Sanity or psychosis is tested by the degree of conjunction or disjunction between two persons where the one is sane by common consent.
>
> The critical test of whether or not a patient is psychotic is a lack of congruity, an incongruity, a clash, between him and me. The 'psychotic' is the name we have for the other person in a disjunctive relationship of a particular kind. It is only because of this disjunction that we start to examine his urine, and look for anomalies in the graphs of the electrical activity of his brain.
>
> (Laing, 1965, p. 36)

It matters how we approach a person, which conditions how we see them and how they act towards us. Sanity and insanity are consensual issues. The clinical examples in *The Divided Self* bring a different view that makes intentional sense or meaning and interpretation for the same phenomena that psychiatrists see as diseased brain function and behavior. Laing liked to quote Robbie Burns: "A men's a man for a' that".

The term 'sanity' goes back through Middle French, 'santé' (health), and further back to Latin: 'sanus', 'sound', 'healthy'. It meant the ability to flourish as a whole person, both mentally and physically. Insanity involves being impeded by oneself, even if others influence that blocking. This is more global than distress and particular neurotic behaviors.

Etymologically, sanity has a sense of appropriateness, of wholeness, of robustness. Healing has sense of health or wholeness. This has a sense of being able to deal with the environment, other people, what presents itself to be in an optimal condition to work and love.

Laing did not have a theory of sanity as such. Just as Freud didn't have a theory of normality, but rather of neurosis. Laing's emphasis was on mental distress and its relation to insanity.

Laing regarded himself as practicing along the mainstream line over time of the humanistic tradition of medicine. As the interviews with Bob Mullan confirm, Laing saw himself, at least clinically, as a 'conservative revolutionary', involving a revolution that brings in the old values. He identified with the 'older humanitarian clinicians' who saw patients under their care and protection and were sceptical of the new modes of automatic medications, electric shock and lobotomies. Early in his career in the army and psychiatry and neurology wards, he recalled that when he was asked to consult, 'the expression they would use would be – "Well, Ronnie's very conservative"' (Mullan, 1995, p. 107). Conservatism in Laing's case in this context means not abandoning some fundamental precepts handed down through the western tradition in particular, together with being socially libertarian, respecting individual choice.

Indeed, Laing was like a nineteenth-century humanist who saw that humans were agents and not necessarily beyond all reason. Instead, he thought it was necessary to reframe and extend the concept of reason in a similar fashion to how Freud reframed and teased out the consequences of the ego not being master in its own house. That, I think, was an important part of the attraction of Freud, whom Laing considered to be a hero of the underworld (Laing, 1965, p. 25).

Respect for the agency of the patient is a critical value in its own right here – that is to optimize their rights and abilities to make their own decisions and to see a decision made for another person as inferior to a decision that the person makes himself or herself, even if it is the same decision! That is, there is a premium in the liberal Enlightenment tradition of *autonomy* that I believe Laing taps into. On an individual level, I can have authority over my actions. On a collective level, we can say, as Jean-Jacques Rousseau suggests, that democracy is better than other systems not simply because of its generally better results, but because it is in an important sense 'ours'. We own it in principle. With Descartes's *'Cogito ergo sum'*, 'I think therefore I am', modern philosophy begins with the individual. It continued into the Enlightenment with natural and inalienable rights, social contracts rooted in the individual and then came to be a default emphasis starting from the individual and siding with him or her, sceptical of the inroads of religion, the state or the collective. Methodological individualism, begins with the individual and how they see the world and their choices. Methodological collectivist approaches from Durkheim and Marx to communism, identity politics and political correctness, assume knowledge of the individual way beyond their choice and experience.

Mill's idea that 'each is his own best judge' is a pretty good default modus operandi. People are good enough in themselves and don't have to be changed by experts or society, and if they are, it is likely to be in the wrong direction. But according to Mill, even if we aren't ideal, it's not only far riskier to take over individual autonomy. It also helps to render us supine and uncreative.

Laing's lecture, 'My Approach to Psychiatry', is particularly germane to his approach to sanity and insanity (Laing, 1977). Unfortunately, the transcript is not publicly available, but I will cite some salient excerpts. The lecture delineates what I consider to be at the heart of Laing's sensibility on these subjects. Now, more than four decades later, for many reasons, including Laing's contributions, I think there is a far more diverse mental health scene despite much mainstream thinking that Laing remained critical of.

Laing speaks in the lecture of our sense of distress when we are in a position of not being able to fend for ourselves and thus fall into the position of 'being at the mercy of other people'. This applies not only to say childbirth or being old and frail but obviously extends to severe mental illness.

Laing confesses to having no solution to the dilemma of how to deal with such interfaces and illustrates it with a vignette about a friend who introduced group therapy into his psychiatric unit. His friend told him the story of a woman with phobias who was prescribed group therapy but couldn't bring herself one morning to go into the therapy room. Laing continues,

> On the contrary, she ran out the door of the ward that was usually shut, and made off down the corridor and was pursued by the staff. She was brought down with a tackle and carried back to the ward, and given an injection, intramuscularly, of tranquiliser. And it acted in about half an hour so that she was able to walk into the group therapy room and participate in the last forty minutes of the group therapy, which she wouldn't have been able to do without that injection. So he was putting to me, 'Well, we give tranquilisers and electric shock if necessary to bring people to the position that they're able to get help from people like you'.

Laing explains:

> I wouldn't have gone after her down the corridor, I wouldn't have ordered injections for her, and so on, He simply says to me. Well, that seems to me that you have abdicated your medical responsibility. . . . This lady is overwhelmed by anxieties which are obviously coming up from her . . . hyperactive midbrain, and you're refusing to give her insulin, as you might give a diabetic. . . . (It would) enable her to be in a state of mind that she wants to be in anyway, such that she can enter the room and participate in group psychotherapy.

Laing cites another example of a seminar with senior psychiatrists where Laing described a scenario in which if he were psychotic, he could be certified, given tranquilizers and electro-shock even if he wasn't doing harm to anyone. Laing regards this as ominous and really frightening. The psychiatrists say he is paranoid. As Laing puts it,

> But that's . . . about as far as . . . the actual dialogue, can go. Because I say I'm absolutely shit-scared at that, and they say I'm paranoid and that's the end of the discussion.

Whenever Laing describes the phenomenological, existential or ontological pre-suppositions behind psychiatric practices, he says,

> Then it all seems to them to be just a lot of nonsense, just a lot of words. And I don't see how to get past that. . . . It doesn't cut any ice with those people who don't accept that such a problematic exists. And it's so easy then for them to say that all of those people who don't necessarily agree with me, but agree that I'm talking about something that concerns them, are all members of some sort of clique or cult, or some sort of walled off peculiar attitude of mind. That's one reason I've objected so much to us collectively and individually being called "anti-psychiatrists". In objecting to this sort of attitude I certainly feel that I'm objecting to it on the basis of the mainstream intellectual Western tradition, not some localised and temporary and transient peculiar queer fashion.
>
> [This tradition] has never allowed us to say that we are simply lumps of physical stock, that when something appears to be the matter with our emotions or our minds or our intentions, our motives and so on, that's not all to be dealt with by a chemical infusion into the body whether we like it or not.

In Laing's view, looking at patients in mental hospitals and their case records makes it *more* obscure and problematic, even about why they are there. Laing says that behind the system is the simple division between natural scientific explanation and the search for intelligibility. 'And it goes all the way into the most organic of conditions'.

Considering patients he had seen in 25 years of clinical practice, Laing says that 'everyone who came to see me voluntarily because they are in a miserable state of distress etc., is frightened.

> And they might be frightened of the sky falling down, or the earth caving in, or being frightened of going out into open spaces, or staying in closed rooms, etc. but the primary fear when it comes to the bit hasn't even got a name for it . . . and it's that people are frightened of other people. You can smell it, the fear that we have of each other. . . . That fear gets some people down perhaps more than others. and they lapse into a state of distress whereby they're unable to hold their own. . . . If you weaken then God help you, and then you're at the mercy of other people. We're proposing that it should not be against the law for people to refuse. It should not be against the law for people to live it out in however a miserable way they may be.

Laing says it comes down to

> [A] . . . civil rights thing that comes to the basic issues of law and order, civic regulation of our conduct between ourself and how we deal with dissent, disagreement and disjunctions between us. And in a wee while this thing is tilted in such a direction we can't really have even a free debate or discussion about

it. . . . Our patients are kidnapped in the street by the police, and taken off to mental hospitals, given tranquilisers and electric shocks that *they* don't want, that *we* don't want them to have, that the people that are living with them don't want them to have, because the hospital thinks that that's what they *ought* to have, because they're diagnosed as catatonic, or hypophrenic, and there's no counter to that.

Laing concludes the lecture by saying, 'We're leaving them alone' and asked for people 'to realise the enormity of the power that is wielded and to accept the principle of live and let live' (Laing, 1977).

This fits the syndrome which Laing described as the imposition of 'knowledge without love'. The liberal principle enunciated by John Stuart Mill goes beyond any utilitarian view that the expert intervention, even if unwanted, produces better results and that the freedom to choose is an important value in its own right.

Part of what may underlie the importance of the value of freedom to choose may be some protection from the fear of being at the mercy of others who are untrustworthy strangers, those not known but that may need to be relied upon. If familiars – family and friends – are scary enough, how much more frightening might strangers be? To function in any stable way, it has been found that any social group larger than a small village of around 150 people needs to make arrangements to deal with strangers, people who are not personally known to everybody.

I imagine that if the underlying role of primary fear of being at the mercy of others is taken into account, the pleasure quotient and results of the system might be far lower in utilitarian terms than is assumed. Intervention in this sense could be somewhat counterproductive, reinforcing the very fear that it is aimed at combatting. Fear and its consequences need to be factored into the equation.

In his classic essay, 'Two Concepts of Liberty', historian of ideas Sir Isaiah Berlin made a very useful distinction when he outlined freedom as having two quite differing and conflicting aspects, which he termed 'positive' and 'negative' freedom, 'freedom to' and 'freedom from' (Berlin, 1969).

The exponents of positive freedom, from Plato to totalitarians such as communists and Nazis, assume that the state based upon knowledge or ideology would know better than the individual how it is best to live and would organize society along the lines of what is seen as best for everyone. Not just Plato but totalitarians believe in such a general perspective.

Clearly, for example, Karl Marx is a proponent of positive freedom. In Marx's view, individual rights are secondary, and people become truly free only with the construction of a perfect classless society. Freedom is the fulfillment of human nature and involves changing people by changing society. Like Mill and, in a different way, Soren Kierkegaard, Laing's starting point is the individual and their experience. It is a methodological individualist approach rather than a methodological collectivist approach that begins with the collective and situates the individual within that context.

Such a collectivist systemic perspective provides a perfect excuse for controlling individuals. And if Laing was allergic to anything, it was the risk and the reality of coercion of self by others when there is no threat. On the other hand, negative freedom, 'freedom from', is paradigmatically represented by the philosophy of John Stuart Mill. Mill emphasizes that the state keeps out of individual's affairs beyond the minimum, individual rights and the right of people not to be deliberately harmed. People should be able to do what they like within the law. There is faith in individuals and their actions and mistrust of the state and being dependent upon it, as it puts them at risk of being harmed by it or simply because people are their own best judges.

Obviously, the state has grown enormously since Mill's day, and many of the real benefits of modern civilization depend on a welfare state, detailed regulations and controls, adequate defense, etc. However, a balance is needed – society needs to be preserved from the tyranny of the majority perhaps at least as much as it needs to be organized for them.

Moreover, respect for the individual means more than just allowing them space. The positive approach is a belief in the creativity of human agents and their potential for flourishing in their own way and cultivating optimal socio-cultural and economic conditions for this to be able to occur. The good is not just a quantitative hedonic subtraction experiment of the feelings of pleasure minus the feelings of pain. Instead, as Aristotle suggested, the good lies not in the criterion of a sense of pleasure, but in the variety in the state of the fulfilment of a range of diverse goals. Diversity and variety are significant values in their own right.

Laing's approach about how we treat people called sane and insane echoes John Stuart Mill's description of the goals of his essay, *On Liberty:*

The sole end for which mankind are warranted, individually or collectively, in interfering with the liberty of action of any of their number, is self-protection. That the only purpose for which power can be rightfully exercised over any member of a civilized community, against his will, is to prevent harm to others. His own good, either physical or moral, is not a sufficient warrant. He cannot rightfully be compelled to do or forbear because it will be better for him to do so, because it will make him happier, because, in the opinions of others, to do so would be wise, or even right. . . . The only part of the conduct of any one, for which he is amenable to society, is that which concerns others. In the part which merely concerns himself, his independence is, of right, absolute. Over himself, over his own body and mind, the individual is sovereign.

(Mill, 1859 [2002], Chapter 1)

If the patients do no harm to anyone else, they should not be coerced for their own good. There is a sense of tolerance and respect for the diversity of living, and it begins with the assumption that different people's actions and behaviours might make some sense in terms of their agency.

This means that there isn't so much a positive picture of what a sane person is, but instead a view that the term 'insane' starts with the individual and doesn't need to generalize and factor the person out.

Furthermore, as the Nobel Prize winner Freidrich Hayek (1948) argues in the realm of economics, human beings are not intelligent enough for the central planning involved with socialism. Too many variables are involved in interactions with one another for central planning to be effective. According to Hayek, our knowledge is too limited to generate and organize collective resources through collective command authority. Evidence for this is not hard to find. I need go no further than to cite the comment by Richard Horton, editor of the prestigious British medical journal, *The Lancet:*

> The case against science is straightforward: in scientific literature, perhaps half, may simply be untrue. Afflicted by studies with small sample sizes, tiny effects, invalid exploratory analyses, and flagrant conflicts of interest, together with an obsession for pursuing fashionable trends of dubious importance, science has taken a turn towards darkness.
>
> (Horton, 2015)

From pharmaceutical companies, to individual scientists and academics, to governments, to departments seeking funding, to journals and universities and the media, everybody is structurally incentivized in the wrong direction to fix this mess. So obviously *caveat emptor* needs to be the rule, and scepticism and criticism of assumptions, not groupthink, needs to rule in going back to basics. Since nobody can truly guarantee that the experts, the authorities, 'those who know', really do know, we are better off with default conditions for robust debate and critical inquiry. This needs to be in the context of maximum individual and private freedom of expression and action compatible with not harming others and social order. The prevalence of what Laing terms 'knowledge without love' assumes a knowledge that may be questioned today more than ever. I don't think that there is as much agreed-upon fact or knowledge as is claimed or assumed today in science or beyond. Although there is a lot of groupthink in our globalized, interconnected and instant-communications world, many claims to knowledge are still contested. With questioning of the truth of claims to knowledge, we could even find ourselves in a situation of 'knowledge without knowledge'.

So even on the grounds of utility alone, coercion in one's own best interests could often be counterproductive since we can't trust the experts, who might be wrong anyway. And if somebody is right and prevents debate because it is right (e.g., the Earth being round), then, as Mill argued, we risk ceasing to utilize our critical capacity and become dogmatic and complacent, which leads to further errors and less creativity.

A utilitarian has no problem in principle with interference with individual freedom, if it really works for his or her own good. Often each may be their own best judge by default, as they control and know their own domain best. But in the case of mentally ill people, utilitarians could argue that they have ceded this knowledge and apprehension to others who are experts about the body or the brain and are not out of their minds.

Considering the unreliability of science and expertise and claims to knowledge, Mill's principle 'Each is their own best judge' may well be the best bet even as a statement of pragmatism and utility. But for Mill, it is far more than that as a principle in itself. And I think that is very much so for Laing.

For Laing, the approach of the modern medical/psychiatric profession is essentially utilitarian and too often leaves out our personal involvement. In fact, 'evidence-based medicine' is clearly utilitarian in all senses of the term. It facilitates the best interests of the patient in their own expert minds, using a pragmatic approach, but leaves out the core issue about who decides. There is nothing wrong with evidence, but we need to always consider what counts as evidence, especially when it comes to psychology and psychiatry. Moreover, times have changed to a more consumer-focused society today.

Laing adopts a longer view. Overall, he inserted his ideas into the great chain of philosophical inquiries into the nature of humans and how we can best relate with others. He saw the greatest fear as the legitimate fear of other people who must earn our trust. This was very much in the conservative humanistic tradition of Edmund Burke and John Stuart Mill and, of course, Freud.

Laing asks us to notice, to recognize and insert another dimension, level or layer into what is happening in cases of prima facie insanity, to insert a question mark between their stimulus and our response. According to the Laing of *The Divided Self*, insane people may deny their own agency by treating themselves as things.

Whatever the truth of such a large generalization, it is vital that practitioners are mindful and careful not to miss the quality of the patient's agency by treating them as akin to mechanisms. This involves the evocation of primary fear of other people that can be easily missed if the patient is not viewed as an agent. It's reframing, perhaps deframing, depending on the glasses we wear. If you don't look, you don't see. This is another example of Laing's concept of 'the obvious', that which stands in front of us that we don't see. It requires respect for experience without being a slave to it. It requires a particular sensibility, the kind that Laing naturally had when meeting schizophrenics in the back wards of Gartnavel Royal Mental Hospital in Glasgow early in his career.

Laing helped many things to change within psychiatry and psychology and alerted us to many fundamental pitfalls. It remains important today to keep an open mind and a nuanced approach that includes drugs and other aids to best treat people termed insane. Laing reminds us that this needs to be at least as much art as science, the assertions of which are often not validated anyway, and requires continued care and mindfulness. Laing points to the importance of context in understanding and explaining throughout his work. This implies that there are no general answers about how to deal with specific situations. One size does not fit all. Furthermore, a rulebook for diagnosis and treatment can give the impression of certainty when there is so much ambiguity, complexity and uncertainty in actual clinical situations.

Moreover, human development and healthy living, particularly in infancy, childhood and old age, involve a necessary and healthy dependence on others. Responsibility develops over time and is not cut and dried. Where and when do we draw the line except pragmatically? The many faces of fear can be boiled down to fear of dependence on others because of the risk that they might harm us. If hell is other people, as Sartre proposed, heaven is other people too. Principles of 'live and let live' involve also cultivation, care and love beyond leaving people to their own devices. The Judeo-Christian tradition, in which Laing was schooled and enthusiastic about, as well as other world traditions, treat people as moral agents intrinsically valuable and deserving of respect. Laing raises crucial questions about the complex knots involved in so many of our taken-for-granted approaches.

References

Berlin, I. (1969). Two concepts of liberty. In *Four essays on liberty*, pp. 118–172. Oxford: Oxford University Press.

Hayek, F. (1948). *Individualism and economic order*. Chicago: University of Chicago Press.

Horton, R. (2015). Offline: What is medicine's 5 sigma? *The Lancet*, 11. https://doi.org/10.1016/S0140-6736(15)60696-1

Kirsner, D. (1990). Across an abyss: Laing, Jaspers and Sartre. *Journal of the British Society for Phenomenology*, 21: 209–216.

Laing, R. D. (1965). *The divided self: An existential study in sanity and madness*. Harmondsworth: Penguin Books (Original edition 1960).

Laing, R. D. (1977). My approach to psychiatry. *Transcript of lecture*. London, May 24. Unpublished.

Mill, J. S. (1859 [2002]). *On liberty*. New York: Dover.

Mullan, R. (1995). *Mad to be normal: Conversations with R. D. Laing*. London: Free Association Books.

Chapter 3

Sanity and the State of the World

Fritjof Capra, PhD

Fifty years ago, R. D. Laing famously said:

> Insanity – a perfectly rational adjustment to an insane world.
> In *The Politics of Experience* Laing expanded on this radical idea (see Laing, 1967):

> The condition of alienation, of being asleep, of being unconscious, of being out of one's mind, is the condition of the normal man. Society highly values its normal man. It educates children to lose themselves and to become absurd, and thus to be normal. Normal men have killed perhaps 100 million of their fellow normal men in the last fifty years.

In this essay, I would like to reflect on the current state of the world and to discuss some of the characteristics of our modern society, which Laing, with great prescience, identified as symptoms of insanity half a century ago.

Interconnectedness of World Problems

When we look at the state of the world today, what is most evident is the fact that the major problems of our time – energy, environment, climate change, poverty – cannot be understood in isolation. They are systemic problems, which means that they are all interconnected and interdependent (see Capra and Luisi, 2014, p. 362ff.). As Pope Francis (2015) puts it in his remarkable encyclical "Laudato Sì":

> Our common home is falling into serious disrepair. . . . [This is] evident in large-scale natural disasters as well as social and even financial crises, for the world's problems cannot be analyzed or explained in isolation. . . . It cannot be emphasized enough how everything is interconnected.

Unfortunately, this realization has not yet dawned on most of our political and corporate leaders who are unable to "connect the dots," to use a popular phrase. Instead of taking into account the interconnectedness of our major problems, their

DOI: 10.4324/9781003564294-4

so-called "solutions" tend to focus on a single issue, thereby simply shifting the problem to another part of the system – for example, by producing more energy at the expense of biodiversity, public health, or climate stability.

From a psychiatric point of view, this failure to see things in context is seen as a neurotic state and is described with terms like dissociation, isolation, or compartmentalization. It is, indeed, a very general symptom of insanity.

Moreover, our leaders refuse to recognize how their piecemeal solutions affect future generations. They may refer to "sustainable development," which in itself is a problematic term, but they lack any intergenerational responsibility. So we have dissociation from the wider context of today's problems, if you wish, in space and in time.

The lack of concern about the future, fueled by materialism and greed, is a typical symptom of a manic state. The Greeks called it "hubris" and illustrated it with the legend of the "Midas touch," in which King Midas turns everything he touches into gold at his own detriment.

The Illusion of Perpetual Growth

The fundamental dilemma underlying our major global problems seems to be the illusion that unlimited growth is possible on a finite planet. This irrational belief in perpetual economic growth amounts to a clash between linear thinking and the nonlinear patterns in our biosphere – the ecological networks and cycles that constitute the web of life. This highly nonlinear global network contains countless feedback loops through which the planet balances and regulates itself. Our current economic system, by contrast, does not seem to recognize any limits.

It's not only that corporate CEOs, like those of the big oil companies or the big pharmaceutical companies, prefer short-term profits to facing the long-term consequences. That itself is immoral. But the situation is worse, because this irrational belief in perpetual growth on a finite planet is shared by virtually all academic and corporate economists, who have integrated it into their so-called "scientific" economic models.

In psychiatric terms, we are dealing here with a severe case of delusion, a symptom of serious mental illness. Combined with the manic desire for ever more money and power, it often results in a persistent denial of reality. Let me give you an example. Today we know the amount of carbon dioxide that we can still emit into the atmosphere by mid-century while staying below the limit beyond which climate change is likely to spin out of control. It is a very large number – 565 gigatons! But it is only 20 percent of the proven coal and oil reserves of the fossil fuel companies and oil-producing states. In other words, in order to avoid total climate collapse, the energy corporations need to leave 80 percent of their reserves in the ground.

Rather than do that, these companies plan to extract and burn all of their reserves and, in fact, they continually explore for new oil reserves. In other words, wrecking the planet is an integral part of their business plans. To justify their actions, they systematically deny the science of climate change. In fact, they finance sophisticated disinformation campaigns to mislead the public about the nature and severity of the climate crisis. All this adds up to a pathological denial of reality.

Global Capitalism

Economic and corporate growth are the driving forces of global capitalism, the dominant economic system today. In this global economy, capital works in real time, moving rapidly through global financial networks. From these networks, it is invested in all kinds of economic activity, and most of what is extracted as profit is channeled back into the meta-network of financial flows. Sophisticated information and communication technologies enable financial capital to move rapidly from one option to another in a relentless global search for investment opportunities.

The dual role of computers as tools for rapid processing of information and for sophisticated mathematical modeling has led to the virtual replacement of gold and paper money by ever more abstract financial products – "future options," "hedge funds," "derivatives," and so on. The end result of all these technological and financial innovations has been the transformation of the global economy into a giant, electronically operated casino. Accordingly, the operations of these new financial markets have become known as "casino finance."

At the existential human level, the most alarming feature of the new economy may be that it is shaped in very fundamental ways by machines. The so-called "global market," strictly speaking, is not a market at all, but a network of machines programmed according to a single value – money-making for the sake of making money – to the exclusion of all other values. In other words, the global economy has been designed in such a way that all ethical dimensions are excluded.

What we see in this global capitalism is a flight from the real world to an extreme level of abstraction. Politics today is largely shaped by economics and, in particular, by Goldman Sachs and the other big investment banks on Wall Street. Their economists are mesmerized by blips of numbers on Wall Street's electronic tickers, and the so-called "health" of these gigantic banks is more important to the world's politicians than the well-being of actual individuals and communities. So, again, we have a loss of contact with reality and endless permutations of multiple levels of abstraction, which is typical, for example, in the writings of schizophrenics.

Self-Destruction

To repeat, at the center of the global economy we find a network of financial flows, which has been designed without any ethical framework. In fact, social inequality and social exclusion are inherent features of economic globalization, widening the gap between the rich and the poor and increasing world poverty.

In this economic system, perpetual growth is pursued relentlessly by promoting excessive consumption and a throw-away economy that is energy and resource intensive, generating waste and pollution and depleting the Earth's natural resources. Moreover, these environmental problems are exacerbated by global climate change, caused by our energy-intensive and fossil fuel–based technologies, and threatening the very survival of human civilization.

Today, we are the only species that is destroying its own habitat and, in doing so, causing mass extinctions of countless other species. Indeed, violence against ourselves and against others is an outstanding characteristic of our society, especially in the United States, where we can witness an epidemic of economic, military, and police violence. And violence, against oneself and others, is, of course, one of the primary symptoms of insanity. A collective, albeit unconscious, suicidal tendency has also been suggested.

Qualitative Growth

So, what are we to do? How can we restore sanity? It seems that our key challenge is to shift from an economic system based on the notion of unlimited growth to one that is both ecologically sustainable and socially just. "No growth" is not the answer. Growth is a central characteristic of all life; but growth in nature is not linear, and neither is it unlimited. While certain parts of organisms, or ecosystems, grow, others decline, releasing and recycling their components, which become resources for new growth.

This kind of balanced, multifaceted growth is well known to biologists and ecologists. I call it "qualitative growth" to contrast it with the concept of quantitative growth, measured in terms of the undifferentiated index of the gross domestic product, the GDP, used by today's economists (see Capra and Henderson, 2009). In fact, most of what is called "growth" today is waste, which means that we have an economics of largely waste and destruction.

Qualitative growth, by contrast, is growth that enhances the quality of life through generation and regeneration. In living organisms, ecosystems, and societies, qualitative growth includes an increase of complexity, sophistication, and maturity.

Instead of assessing the state of the economy in terms of the crude quantitative measure of GDP, we need to qualify growth, i.e., we need to distinguish between "good" growth and "bad" growth and then increase the former at the expense of the latter.

From the ecological point of view, the distinction between "good" and "bad" economic growth is obvious. Bad growth is growth of production processes and services that externalize social and environmental costs, are based on fossil fuels, involve toxic substances, deplete our natural resources, and degrade the Earth's ecosystems. Good growth is growth of more efficient production processes and services that involve renewable energies, zero emissions, continual recycling of natural resources, and restoration of the Earth's ecosystems.

Systemic Solutions

Qualitative growth means growth of a living system, not at the expense of other living systems, but within the context of their own qualitative growth. In other words, qualitative growth naturally involves systemic solutions – solutions to problems within the context of other problems.

Over the last few decades, the research institutes and centers of learning of the global civil society have developed and proposed hundreds of such systemic solutions all over the world. Here is just one example of a typical systemic solution in the area of agriculture. If we changed from our chemical, large-scale industrial agriculture to organic, community-oriented, sustainable farming, this would contribute significantly to solving three of our biggest problems. (1) It would greatly reduce our energy dependence, because we are now using one-fifth of our fossil fuels to grow and process food. (2) The healthy, organically grown food would have a huge positive effect on public health, because many chronic diseases – heart disease, stroke, diabetes, and so on – are linked to our diet. And (3), organic farming would contribute significantly to fighting climate change, because an organic soil is a carbon-rich soil, which means that it draws CO_2 from the atmosphere and locks it up in organic matter. It is worth noting that today, carbon sequestration in soil and plants is the only known and proven strategy that can remove carbon from the atmosphere and, over time, reduce the atmospheric concentration of CO_2.

In my textbook, coauthored with Pier Luigi Luisi, we review a wide variety of such systemic solutions in detail (see Capra and Luisi, 2014, p. 394ff.). They include proposals to reshape economic globalization and restructure corporations; new forms of ownership that are not extractive but generative; a wide variety of systemic solutions to the interlinked problems of energy, food security, poverty, and climate change; and finally, the large number of systemic design solutions known collectively as ecodesign. Together, these systemic solutions provide compelling evidence that today we have the knowledge and the technologies to build a sustainable future. What we need is political will and leadership. In other words, the core problem is not conceptual or technical. It is a problem of ethics.

As the Czech playwright and statesman Václav Havel famously put it, what we need most urgently to solve our global problems is a "moral compass." This is also the message that R. D. Laing tried to convey again and again. I well remember a conversation about science and consciousness Laing and I had in 1980 (see Capra, 1988, pp. 138–139), during which he told me:

> The new science, the new epistemology, has got to be predicated upon a change of heart, upon a complete turning around; from the intent to dominate and control nature to the idea of, for example, Francis of Assisi, that the whole creation is our companion, if not our mother. That is part of your turning point. Only then can we address ourselves to alternative perceptions that will come into view.

References

Capra, F. (1988). *Uncommon wisdom*. New York: Simon and Schuster.

Capra, F. and Henderson, H. (2009). *Qualitative growth in outside insights*. London: Institute of Chartered Accountants in England and Wales.

Capra, F. and Luisi, P. L. (2014). *The systems view of life*. New York: Cambridge University Press.

Laing, R. D. (1967). *The politics of experience*. New York: Ballantine.

Pope Francis (2015). *Laudato Si'*. Vatican: Libreria Editrice Vaticana.

II

What Is Therapeutic?

Chapter 4

On Sympathy

The Role of Love in the Therapeutic Encounter

M. Guy Thompson, PhD

Of all the words that we use as a matter of course in our daily lives, love is probably the most difficult to define or grasp. I have yet to meet anyone, no matter how wise or worldly, who claims to know precisely what love is. Yet even if no one understands it, there is little doubt that love in fact exists. For virtually everyone, no matter how rich or poor, crazy or sane, handsome or ugly, has experienced it, both in the passive and active sense of the word. Everyone has loved and been loved, or they wouldn't be human. Yet we have no paucity of opinion as to its effects and, like happiness, we employ all manner of cunning and device to procure it, despite our failure to ever fully possess it. Like a visitor we wish would stay but has other places to go, we reconcile ourselves to its presence on terms we can neither dictate nor control.

It is a matter of common wisdom that we are never more vulnerable, or foolish, than when we are in love with another human being. Our only protection from its artifice is to try our best to defend ourselves against it, by telling ourselves we don't need or want it, or to set our standards so high that no one can possibly meet them. Such strategies are employed regularly by the neurotic, though not without a substantial cost. For what value does life have without it? No matter how much we may deny it, all of us share a common bond that makes us the human creatures we are: *we cannot live without love in one form or other*. No matter how loath we are to admit it, our singular goal in life is to procure as much love as we can get, no matter how successful or futile our efforts may be. Even when we feel without love, our longing persists in the deepest depressions of our being.

The topic of this chapter is to explore the specifically therapeutic aspects of love. This may seem like a futile exercise, and to others perhaps foolish. After all, many therapists today doubt that love plays any role in therapy and, indeed, if and when it manifests its appearance, it may well signal the end of the therapy relationship. This perspective may explain why the word love is seldom invoked when describing the basic elements of the therapeutic process. Sigmund Freud, the inventor of psychotherapy, was also reluctant to sing love's praises in the context of the therapy relationship. Acting on such feelings was strictly forbidden. *Yet it was Freud who was the first to suggest that all neuroses are the consequence of a broken heart*. To suggest that love, or its absence, is capable of driving us crazy doesn't

DOI: 10.4324/9781003564294-6

necessarily imply that it may also heal. Yet in rare moments, Freud acknowledged that love is the key to a successful therapeutic outcome. This, however, was a rare occurrence in the corpus of Freud's writings.[1] Freud's reluctance to employ the word love in both his theoretical and technical papers has been championed by subsequent analysts, virtually all of whom opt to focus instead on the so-called "transference" aspect of the relationship. Even to this day, few analysts realize that this convoluted and much-misunderstood technical term was originally employed by Freud as a synonym for love.

The word love just doesn't sound scientific, does it? More than ever before psychotherapists today seem eager to demonstrate just how scientifically valid their version of psychotherapy is. To suggest that therapy is really about love doesn't further this argument. If anything, it makes the therapeutic dyad sound sentimental, superficial, soft-hearted, and simplistic. And it makes the therapist who dares to invoke this word look foolish, unprofessional, and not well trained. So we come up with all kinds of alternative, scientific-sounding terms in its place, including the just-mentioned transference, as well as the words countertransference, cathexis, sublimation, attachment, and perhaps the most ubiquitous of all, empathy. In fact, most therapists insist that a capacity for empathy is the single most important trait that we can develop as clinicians. My thesis is that empathy, whatever its value, isn't enough. In fact, I want to argue that if therapists focus all their efforts on furthering empathic intuition alone but neglect to embody heartfelt *sympathy*, the results may well border on the grotesque.

Before turning my attention to what I mean by the term sympathy and how it manifests in therapy, I want to say a few words about the other kinds of love that sympathy is sometimes associated with. For the most part, the Greeks spoke about three distinctive kinds of love: *eros*, *philia*, and *agapé*, the last of which is often Latinized as *caritas*, from which we get the English word *charity*, which isn't exactly what *caritas* means.[2] *Eros* is the version of love with which we are most familiar. This is because Freud made it ubiquitous in our lives, arguing that it is operative in virtually all relationships, however intimate or impersonal they may be. Even if Freud is correct in this, the Greeks believed there are higher forms of love than the kind that is explicitly erotic or sexual. What these higher forms of love share in common is that they assume a capacity for self-sacrifice, for putting the other person's needs over our own. Everyone, except for perhaps the craziest person, is conversant with erotic love. But what about *philia*? This is an explicitly non-erotic form of love that the Greeks believed epitomizes friendship, which I have explored in chapter one, as well as elsewhere.[3] Montaigne, for example, suggested that friendship occasions a unique type of love that is necessarily free of sexual interest. R. D. Laing confided to me once that he thought friendship comes closest to embodying the therapeutic relationship. He even proposed that the so-called therapy "patient" or client is essentially a person you sell an hour of your friendship to, like a prostitute might, but without the sex. This is perhaps the reason that sex is antithetical to therapy, because it compromises the subtle forms of self-less compassion that sexual interest abandons.

However, it is the third form of love, *agapé*, that is most relevant to the development of genuine sympathy. This is because *agapé* is by far the most selfless form of love. Meister Eckhart, the fourteenth-century German theologian and mystic, conceived *agapé* as the kind of love we feel for God, which epitomizes Christian love. This is also the specific form of love typically referenced in the Bible. But in place of the Greek term *agapé*, the King James version of the Bible substitutes the Latinized *caritas* instead. Thomas Aquinas, the thirteenth-century Aristotelian theologian, effectively integrated *philia* with *agapé* when he defined charity, or *caritas*, as "a friendship between man and God." He also extended the definition of *caritas* to include the love for one's neighbor, which is just about everyone with whom you come into contact, as well as love for oneself. It was Aquinas's integration of *philia* and *agapé* that helped me entertain the therapeutic relationship as one that is rooted in a special form of love, one that is intrinsically giving, self-effacing, and compassionate, in the Buddhist sense of the word.[4]

So how is all this related to sympathy, and how should we distinguish sympathy from its kissing cousin, empathy? The word sympathy has been so plagiarized by greeting card companies that applying this term to the highest, most selfless love possible may seem trite. But when you take a closer look at the word and its various shades of meaning, I think you will agree that there is no better word in the English language to depict it. Etymologically, both sympathy and empathy derive from the Greek word *pathé* (the same root that gives us "pathology"), which literally means to *feel*, *suffer*, or *experience* something, especially emotions, at the deepest level. All three verbs – to feel, suffer, and experience – are closely intertwined. But whereas empathy denotes the capacity to identify with and essentially intuit what another person is feeling, and even thinking, sympathy entails the ability to *agree with* and so be in harmony with another person's *pathé*. This is why empathy and sympathy are not the same thing, though they ideally complement each other.

I don't think what I'm proposing is something radical or new. The Webster Dictionary, for example, defines empathy as "the ability to share another person's feelings and experiences." Their definition of sympathy is "the feeling that you care about and are sorry about someone else's trouble, grief, or misfortune, a feeling of support for the other person."

This distinction implies that when we sympathize with someone we don't just know or comprehend what they're feeling; we also *feel* what they are feeling *with* them. We suffer *their* suffering, not a facsimile of our own. We resonate with their experience and feel moved by it. This means that we develop a profound affinity for that person. In other words, I am in agreement with, and of *the same mind* as, this person by commiserating with him or her at the deepest, existential level. This isn't a novel idea. After all, Freud was the first analyst to propose that the ideal attitude we should all adopt with our patients is one of "*sympathetic understanding*."

Why sympathetic *understanding* and not just sympathy, full stop? Freud recognized that because infants lack verbal language with which to express their needs, whether they are hungry, wet, or lonely, they rely on their parents to anticipate their needs and intuit what they are. The baby doesn't spell out that she wants to be held, caressed, or nurtured, because she can't. The mother or father, as if by magic, figures it out and provides what is needed. The parent's love for the child plays a central role in this understanding, brought to bear by the extraordinary attention parents bring to the task of parenting. In turn, whenever the infant's needs are understood and met, the infant equates the parent's ability to understand his or her need with love. Children soon learn to equate being understood with *feeling* understood and feeling loved. When we grow up, we seek friends and sexual partners who "understand" us, so to speak. In fact, we all know that nobody is really capable of understanding anyone else. We can't even understand ourselves! What we're really asking for when seeking understanding from a lover, friend, or therapist is a special kind of benevolent, sympathetic *attention.* Freud realized that this is precisely what all of us want from our therapists. This is why it's no accident that the word "therapy," or *therapeia* in Greek, means attention etymologically. It is a form of attention that is, in essence, a gift of love.

Yet sympathy isn't an attitude that one can literally *adopt*, because it cannot be accessed by will. I don't choose to be sympathetic, I succumb to it, naturally, spontaneously, irresistibly. Like the divine interventions the Greeks were so fond of invoking, sympathy, properly speaking, is a *gift of grace.* It spontaneously comes over us and, once felt, holds us in its grip. We have no choice but to feel sympathy whenever it comes over us. When it beckons, we cannot push it aside – nor can we contrive to beckon it on command. Though we cannot control our sympathy, it is anything but blind emotion. Like all emotions, there is an intelligence at work, an intelligence that recognizes the gravity of the other person's situation. Sympathy visits us whenever we feel closest to someone, when we yield to that person's predicament.

In turn, I may express a word of sympathy when someone tells me, for example, that her mother just died. But merely saying the words doesn't guarantee that I genuinely *feel* sympathy. Yet many psychotherapists, especially psychoanalysts, seem loath to use this word or even allude to it in their publications. Instead they opt to talk about *empathy*, as though it is equivalent or even superior to sympathy. As I noted earlier, the word empathy doesn't connote a feeling of love or anything remotely approximating it. To empathize with a patient is essentially a mode of attention that can be developed and perfected, like the act of interpretation. The fact that it may be spontaneous doesn't necessarily imply that it is always heartfelt.

Empathy implies the ability to recognize what the other person is feeling and sometimes thinking, but it is an action of the intellect, not the heart. Its principal vehicle is identification, recognizing something of myself in the other person. Let's take a moment to explore what the psychoanalytic conception of empathy entails, because this is where the concept was first applied to the therapeutic process. For many, it is the psychoanalyst's most cherished technical device.

When I empathize with a person's pain, I have a visceral sense of the pain that person is experiencing. But that's as far as it goes. Empathic attunement doesn't in itself imply compassion. So what are the possible reactions I may experience when I sense anguish in another person? How should I respond? If I don't also feel

sympathy for that person's plight, I am left to ponder what to do with this information. What can I say that may nonetheless prove useful? My mind will race to
connect my patient's experience to my *own* experience, and though this may elicit a
sense of connection with this person, it also tempts me to do something with it. This
is where the danger lies. I may decide that I have to do something more than simply
recognize this person's pain, and in that moment my mind may seize on something
critical to say. Instead of simply sharing the moment and resonating with it, I may
instead urge my patient to take a closer look at that experience, *differently*. Instead
of commiserating with his or her anguish, I may question it. Instead of accepting
my patient's experience, I want to *change* it.

This is often touted as the principal benefit of psychoanalysis – the ability to
look closely at our experience and learn to question our most cherished assumptions. This is indeed a remarkable skill, the same one that is utilized in other disciplines as well, including Buddhism and phenomenology. But this skill can be
deadly if not utilized with compassion, with a heartfelt capacity for *caritas*. Ironically, one of the chief proponents of the use of empathy in psychoanalysis, Heinz
Kohut, arrived at similar conclusions about this concept as I did, but insisted on
referring to sympathy as simply a version of empathy. In his famous inaugural
paper on empathy (first published in 1959), Kohut states that he encountered similar reactions from his patients as the ones I outlined earlier whenever he attempted
to "enlighten" a patient with well-formulated yet critical observations in the form
of incisive interpretations. In the case of his patient, Ms. F, whenever he offered an
interpretation that was not a precise recapitulation of what she had just said, she
became enraged and accused him of "wrecking" her analysis (Kohut, 2011). Once
he stopped accusing Ms. F of resistance, Kohut came to realize that she was teaching him *how to see things exclusively from her point of view*. In other words, once
he stopped trying to reformulate what she was saying from the vantage of a theoretical schema and began to sympathetically listen to her instead, Ms. F felt heard
and understood. She was immediately appreciative of his efforts. Kohut termed this
way of listening *experience-near*.

Kohut also insisted on referring to this ostensibly sympathetic manner of interacting with his patients as a version of *empathy*. I doubt that Kohut was familiar
with Max Scheler's (1954) work on sympathy and so concluded that working from
a more experience-near sensibility was an aspect of empathic attunement. Moreover, nowhere in Kohut's characterization of this process does he acknowledge the
manifestation of love in the relationship. Instead, he refers to invoking empathy as
a strictly "observational" tool that enhances the analyst's capacity for introspection
in the analytic process. I believe this explains why Kohut failed to fully understand
what had been missing in his earlier formulation. *What was missing was the heartfelt feeling of sympathic love for his patient*, not more observational techniques.
Kohut wanted credit for inventing a novel psychoanalytic technique, not for recognizing the ubiquitous role that love plays in therapy. The former is presumably
easier to market than the latter. Kohut even argues it is vital that the analyst, in
adopting this new perspective, *not* completely abandon the more adversarial use of

empathic interpretation. Instead, it should be applied alternately with (sympathetic) experience-near listening in order for the latter to "repair" the damage wrought by the former, instead of employing them simultaneously.

Perhaps one of the lessons we can derive from this is that the practitioner who privileges empathic over sympathic engagement (or, as in Kohut's case, treats them as the same) does so because he overidentifies with the patient. This is the moment when the practitioner's narcissism may leave his (or her) patient in the lurch, when he is more invested in educating his patient than sympathizing with him. Whenever I identify with another person, I perceive that person's experience from the vantage point of my own and so bring myself as well as my intelligence to bear. This is where all the knowledge I have accumulated comes in handy. I have so many ideas, so many possible explanations and theories to call on. This is when my critical faculty comes to the fore, when my mind searches for a way to fix, change, critique, or challenge the other's experience instead of simply *being* with it. Empathy by itself, devoid of a sympathic component, lends itself to working the mind in an intrinsically critical manner. Again, I'm not suggesting there isn't a role for this critical faculty. There most certainly is. There would be no therapy without it. But if this faculty is substituted for sympathy and not guided by it, the consequence can be ugly.

For example, what is it that analysts or therapists are trying to accomplish with their capacity for empathic attunement? How is the mutative element of therapy conceived? It seems to me that the aim of therapy is to engender a capacity for *confiding in one's therapist*, not merely obtaining information, whether conscious or unconscious, by hook or by crook, simply for the sake of divining this or that secret that one's patient isn't yet ready or able to disclose. Kohut is like many analysts who fancy themselves as proficient at getting inside the mind of their patients by divining secrets that may otherwise stay hidden. Harold Searles was also adept at this method.[5] It is as though all that matters to them is knowing stuff, no matter how such knowledge is obtained, smug in the conceit that nothing can ultimately be hidden from them. I don't believe that this kind of regard is therapeutic. It seems to me that what is therapeutic must, on the contrary, derive from developing a modicum of trust that in turn encourages one's patients to share things they have never revealed to anyone else, *when they are ready to do so.*

When I sense that someone I am with, whether a lover, a friend, or a patient, is feeling sad, heartbroken, or lost, I find myself *commiserating* with them. I feel their pain so profoundly and am so affected by it that it may even move me to tears. This isn't empathy. This is *love*. And I suspect that this is why analysts are loath to employ this term and even discourage its role in the therapy process. Analysts don't typically believe that loving one's patients is necessary, appropriate, or desirable. It probably violates one of the many boundaries that analysts seem so eager to erect between themselves and their patients, always at the ready to be proper, correct, professional. I suspect some of them even fear that sympathy may be perilous.

Instead, they see their mission as that of understanding their patients with appropriate detachment but without the sympathetic component that even Freud, the so-called "classical" analyst, advocated. Yes, this cautious and circumspect manner may occasion some measure of concern for the other person, but that isn't the same as loving them.

One of the things I appreciated about my work with R. D. Laing was his emphasis on the specifically spiritual component of love. Despite Laing's notorious preoccupation with the dark side of love, embodied in incidents of deception and subterfuge that sometimes occasion family dynamics (Laing, 1970), Laing believed there is an inherent goodness most people aspire to in their intimate relationships. Notwithstanding Laing's affinity for Eastern disciplines, it was Christianity with which he was most identified. For this reason Kierkegaard (1956, 1995), who was both an existential philosopher and Christian adept, was especially helpful. Laing once told me (1985) that it was from Kierkegaard that he realized the sincerest expression of love is to not "trespass" against others, which is to say to never encroach into someone's personal space. When aspiring to be intimate with another person, he felt it is incumbent on us to do so cautiously, carefully, and, most importantly, tenderly. Though no relationship is free of encroachments, Laing believed that some people are capable of achieving states of communion with others that are relatively free of transgression. *The therapy relationship is explicitly designed to minimize incidents of trespass on another human being. With the possible exception of the clergy, it may very well be the most benign form of relationship that we have ever conceived, explicitly designed to help those most vulnerable.*

Sometimes in his seminars, Laing would read from the Lord's Prayer, inspired, he said, by a book of Aldous Huxley (2009). Laing was especially taken with the part of the prayer that speaks of *trespassing* against one's neighbors and the need to forgive those who trespass against oneself, but especially to forgive one's own trespasses against *them*. Laing seemed particularly sensitive to crossing that line, when therapists, for example, may inadvertently trespass into a space of vulnerability that is not therapeutic, but hurtful. He concluded that some of us are more callous in our conduct with others than we realize. Inspired by Foucault,[6] Laing reckoned that those to whom we entrust ourselves when most vulnerable are oftentimes insensitive to the power they bring to bear when offering help. In his research into families conducted at the Tavistock Institute in the early 1960s, Laing learned that parents are often oblivious when exercising such power, always "for the child's own good." Laing's most controversial message was probably his accusation that the very people who hold themselves out to be helpful – mental health professionals and the like – oftentimes make matters worse by the carelessness they employ with their patients. What they often lack, he suspected, is the requisite sympathy, or *caritas*, with which to treat them. Instead of *caritas*, their patients get "treatment," often of a brutal nature, masquerading as care.

Max Scheler's conception of sympathy (outlined in his major philosophical work, *The Nature of Sympathy* [1954]) exerted a considerable influence on Laing's understanding of the spiritual aspects of love. Like Kierkegaard, Scheler was religious, and much of his philosophical writing was concerned with understanding our relationship with God. Unlike erotic love, which partially blinds us to the other person, sympathy reveals the other person as he or she is, in the most intimate way possible. Scheler was convinced that the only way to truly know another person is through this special manner of regard. This implies that love isn't merely a feeling, but a metaphysical act that brings every aspect of my being to bear when reaching out to another person. *This is why Laing was convinced that sympathy is not merely a way of connecting with a patient who is in pain. It is the most healing component of our work as therapists.* It is love in its essence.

Sympathy is closely related to mercy – both are derivatives of compassion. Anyone who is in a state of distress and seeks help in alleviating it is at the other person's mercy. It implies that the supplicant is defenseless, not in the psychodynamic sense of the term, but simply that one's guard is down, if only momentarily. We ordinarily think of mercy as a sentiment offered to someone who is undeserving of it, as when a criminal asks for clemency. This is different from grace, which is tendered to the deserving. Why *undeserving*, and how is this applicable in the psychotherapy relationship?

It isn't difficult to feel sympathy when moved to tears, but what if a patient becomes hostile and the therapist feels under attack? Ordinarily, a man defends himself against acts of hostility. This is only natural, and more often than not the more prudent reaction. The analyst, however, is expected to *not* respond in kind to expressions of hostility, however much his or her countertransference has been stirred. On the contrary, the analyst is expected to show kindness for his or her patient who, despite the patient's behavior, is nevertheless at the therapist's mercy. Without a genuine *feeling* of mercy, however, no response, no matter how ostensibly proper or circumscribed, will never disguise the underlying resentment or turmoil that the analyst is likely experiencing. Like sympathy, mercy cannot be feigned. If it is not *genuinely experienced*, any ostensibly sympathetic gesture cannot help but fall flat.

Being at the service of one's patients, giving them the kind of attention that no one else can or is willing to, letting them be who they are without judgment, isn't a technique that can be learned. True, it manifests in a job, a job the therapist is paid to perform, so in that sense it's a service. But what we are being paid for isn't to fix something broken or to get someone to see the light that only we possess. What we're really being paid to do is to learn to tolerate the incredibly difficult relationships our patients subject us to, in the most benign way possible.

The only way therapists are able to put up with such tortuous, oftentimes exasperating relationships with people who are neurotic or crazy is to accept them for who they are each and every step of the way. In effect, therapists are expected to care about them, to be patient with them, and to love them, not in the erotic sense, but from a place of *caritas*, which is to say, with genuine sympathy. Contrary to erotic love, the kind of love that seems most helpful in this context is the kind that wants nothing. This means being completely at that person's service, however frustrating, monotonous, or exasperating such service can be.

Despite its elusiveness, our capacity for sympathy is innate. It is one of those things we take for granted, like the water we drink or the air we breathe. Like water and air, we don't do so well without it. In our most intimate relationships, whether lovers, friends, or family, sympathy is the key ingredient that makes them special. We crave sympathy and need it in those moments when our pain is undeniable. Yet we know that we are also capable of losing our sympathy for the very people we love the most. One of the remarkable phenomena I have noticed among some of the couples I have worked with was the absence of sympathy in their marital relationship. One of the first signs that a marriage is on the rocks is the loss of sympathy that one or both of the partners feels for the other's suffering. Each is so preoccupied with his or her own pain that there is little sympathy for that of the partner. In any close relationship, each expects sympathy from the other and is acutely aware when it is missing. Whenever we complain about our jobs, our health, even the weather, to another person, the first thing we look for is an expression of sympathetic commiseration for what we have to put up with. It is the salve that keeps us going despite all the hardships we experience daily. It always improves my mood when I succeed in eliciting it, because its expression confirms that the person who offers it cares about me and regards me with a loving disposition. Yet like erotic desire, sympathy cannot be aroused on command. You feel it or you don't.

If sympathy is so important to us, if we crave and expect it in virtually all of our relationships, then why does it break down? Why withhold it when it is asked of us, when it epitomizes the love we feel for that person? Why are we unable to *feel* sympathy whenever we're called upon to offer it, even with our patients? There are many possible reasons, but perhaps the most common is that the person soliciting sympathy is no longer credible to me. In order to arouse sympathy, one's pain has to be sincere and without guile; it cannot be faked. If I sense that your pain is genuine, I am more likely to feel sympathy for you than if I sense it is not. If I suspect your expression of suffering is contrived, that you are orchestrating the pain you telegraph to me in order to elicit sympathy, then you will lose your credibility with me, and with that credibility you will lose my sympathy. *I can love a person sympathetically only if and when that person is being genuine or authentic with me, which is to say, so long as I believe them.*

This can be a two-edged sword. We may be so desperate for sympathy that we contrive to solicit it by feigning illness, even becoming ill, in the guise of this or that somatic symptom. Freud believed that all our psychological symptoms are the consequence of feeling love-sick. It's a short step from feeling unloved, to feeling sick about it, to asking a therapist for a sympathetic ear. We have known for millennia that for the most part it is the physician's *sympathetic attention* that does the healing, not the treatment itself. Sometimes we are obliged to contrive an illness in order to eventually admit to ourselves that all we really wanted was a little love.

Freud once offered that psychoanalysis is a "cure through love" (see Thompson, 1998). This observation is easy to misconstrue, but he was right. Psychotherapy is a cure through love in a double sense. First, it is imperative that the patient comes to love the therapist, not erotically, but from the perspective of *philia*, like the crucial friend[7] with whom one shares everything. Second, the analyst must also come to love the patient, but not, strictly speaking, as a friend. The therapist may be a friend to her patient, but the patient will never be a friend to the therapist, nor can he. Their relationship is too inequitable, too asymmetrical for a conventional friendship, which needs to be rooted in reciprocity to flourish. The kind of love therapists feel for their patients can only be rooted in *sympathy*, a selfless giving over to the person who the patient happens to be, a person that the therapist is able to cherish for as long as necessary. The love proffered is selfless because therapists don't need their patients to love them in the same way their patients need to feel loved by their therapist. Patients need to be loved because that is what finally, if surreptitiously, heals them. Love is magical that way. Without it, we feel lost.

Finally, therapists need sympathy too. But they aren't likely to get it from their patients! More likely they will get it from their partners, their colleagues, and their own therapists. They may even get it from themselves.

Notes

1 See my "Manifestations of Transference: Love, Friendship, Rapport" (1998) for more on Freud's positive statements to this issue.
2 Charity: benevolence, giving. *Caritas*: the ultimate perfection of the human soul, derived from *agapé* – divine love; the absolute requirement for happiness, man's highest effort. *Caritas* entails love of god, love of one's neighbor, and love of oneself; it is a composite of *agapé* and *eros*. Genuine self-love is rooted in sympathy.
3 See Chapter 5 in my *The Ethic of Honesty*, (2004); Chapter 6 in my *The Death of Desire*, (2016); and Chapter 1 of this volume, my essay on friendship.
4 The etymological roots of the words sympathy and compassion derive from the same roots: the Greek term *pathé*, meaning passion, suffering, emotion. To feel sympathy or compassion is to *be with* one's *pathé*.
5 See the video presentation, *Approaches* (1976), featuring Harold Searles and R. D. Laing, each interviewing in turn a woman who had been hospitalized for depression, for Searles's uncanny ability to intuit information that the woman interviewed was not verbalizing.
6 Foucault was a dear friend of Laing's and resonated with Laing's sensitivity to power dynamics in families as well as society. Virtually all of Foucault's works were in some way or another concerned with the currency of power in human relationships, but an especially telling and useful work was a collection of interviews and essays published in 1980.
7 See (Thompson, 2004, pp. 79–94) for a critique of Masud Kahn's conception of crucial friendship in the transference relationship.

References

Foucault, M. (1980). *Power/knowledge: Selected interviews and other writings, 1972–1977.* New York: Vintage.

Huxley, A. (2009). *The perennial philosophy.* New York and London: Harper Perennial Modern Classics.

Kierkegaard, S. (1956). *Purity of heart is to will one thing: Spiritual preparation for the office of confession* (Douglas V. Steere, Trans.). New York: Harper Torchbooks.

Kierkegaard, S. (1995). *Works of love* (Howard V. Hong and Edna H. Hong, Trans.). Princeton: Princeton University Press.

Kohut, H. (1959). Introspection, empathy, and psychoanalysis – an examination of the relationship between mode of observation and theory. *Journal of the American Psychoanalytic Association*, 7: 459–483.

Kohut, H. (2011). *The search for the self, volume 3: Selected writings of Heinz Kohut 1978–1981*. London: Karnac Books.

Laing, R. D. (1970). *Knots*. London: Tavistock.

Laing, R. D. (1985). Personal communication.

Scheler, M. (1954). *The nature of sympathy* (Peter Heath, Trans.). London: Routledge and Kegan Paul.

Thompson, M. Guy (1998). Manifestations of transference: Love, friendship, rapport. *Contemporary Psychoanalysis*, 34, no. 4: 457–481.

Thompson, M. Guy (2004). *The ethic of honesty: The fundamental rule of psychoanalysis*, pp. 79–94. Amsterdam and New York: Rodopi.

Thompson, M. Guy (2016). *The death of desire: An existential study in sanity and madness*, pp. 121–142. London and New York: Routledge.

Chapter 5

Laing's Conception of Therapy

Douglas Kirsner, PhD

This chapter explores the major themes of Laing's approach to what is therapeutic. Laing was a psychiatrist who trained with the British Psychoanalytic Society as a psychoanalyst and worked and researched at the Tavistock Clinic during the 1960s. His best work was clearly during the 1960s and his many personal difficulties, including alcoholism, impacted on his life and work thereafter.

I see Laing as embarked upon a journey that begins with writing *The Divided Self*, which he drafted by 1956 and published in 1960. It goes way beyond it during the 1960s. His work developed from existential approaches to madness in an individual, to understanding the social and familial politics and context, to theories of communication, and expanded later to encompass spiritual dimensions. Laing had a rare gift for communicating with very disturbed patients and crossing disciplinary boundaries and the ability to communicate difficult questions and concepts in plain language.

Laing delves further into the significance of interactions across several crucial areas: families and ordered patterns of communication, the interactions between therapists and patients, and the nature of the mystifications and confusions that set everyone off course.

For Laing psychotherapy is based on the etymological origin of the term 'therapy' as 'attentiveness'. As Laing told Bob Mullan, 'the name of the game is cultivating tactful attention to each other, *attentiveness*. So, I'm offering my attention and my response in my judgement of what is appropriate, of how to respond to you. I'll be attentive to you' (Mullan, 1995, p. 320). Laing declares, 'They've had my company, my attention, my *engagement* on their behalf' (Mullan, 1995, p. 328). 'A lot of people who have come to see me have said that the main thing they have got from me is that I listen to them' (Mullan, 1995, p. 331). Laing applied Freud's innovation of listening, at least with a wide range of neurotics.

Although Laing made numerous statements about the nature of psychotherapy over the decades, his comment in *The Politics of Experience* (1967) represents his general approach:

> Psychotherapy consists in the paring away of all that stands between us, the props, masks, roles, lies, defenses, anxieties, projections and introjections, in

DOI: 10.4324/9781003564294-7

short, all the carry-overs from the past, transference and counter-transference, that we use by habit and collusion, wittingly or unwittingly, as our currency for relationships.

(p. 39)

According to Laing, 'Psychotherapy must remain *an obstinate attempt of two people to recover the wholeness of being human through the relationship between them*' (Laing, 1967b, p. 45, original emphasis). That said, Laing saw psychotherapy as really an individual endeavour with no particular technique. I once asked him why there wasn't a Laingian school even though he was so famous. He told me that he thought this was because there was no 'Laingian technique', like say a Rogerian, Gestalt, or Freudian approach.

For Laing, psychotherapy is based on the bedrock assumption of who we are as persons, not what we are as mechanisms. For Laing, we are essentially intentional agents involved in praxis rather than resultants of processes. If we look at somebody as a person, we see them differently when viewing them as a complex machine. *The Divided Self* describes what it would be like to bring a *science of persons* described in thoroughgoing personal and internally consistent experiential terms to understand normal and particularly seemingly pathological behaviour and experience. Terms such as 'ontological security', 'engulfment', and 'petrification' explain them in a new way that depends on people being embodied subjects, agents exercising choice, intention, meaning, and experience. Existential terms are the appropriate ones for clinical pictures of human beings. The long-standing debate about whether psychoanalysis and psychoanalytic psychotherapy are natural science or hermeneutic can be somewhat averted by arguing, as the American psychoanalytic researcher George Klein did, that psychoanalysis is in fact two theories in one – the clinical theory, which is largely understandable in terms of intention, meaning, and interpretation resting directly upon clinical data, experience, subjectivity and behaviour, and a meta-psychology, which is at a remove and is cast in the language of natural science. Laing was concerned that much of modern thinking was in the natural science tradition of Descartes and Galileo. Modern physics began with a sharp distinction between the observer and the observed object. However, as Laing suggests,

Any technique concerned with the other without the self, with behaviour to the exclusion of experience, with the relationship to the neglect of the persons in relation, with the individuals to the exclusion of their relationship, and most of all, with an object-to-be changed rather than a person-to-be-accepted, simply perpetuates the disease it purports to cure. . . . Our concern is with the origins of experience in relation.

(Laing, 1967, p. 45)

Laing describes the possibility of psychotic behaviour as potentially more intelligible than was normally described in psychiatry, though I believe he over-reached in appearing to describe schizophrenic behaviour and experience in *The Divided Self* along the same lines as Sartre's concept of self-deception and later in *The Politics of Experience* adopting a different tack, describing schizophrenia as a potentially healing voyage of discovery. The impact of other people and their perceptions became of increasing importance for Laing as he moved from self to self-other interactions, to the family, beyond to the social world, and then to the cosmos in weaving webs of meta, meta-meta-perceptions, and so on that produce immense, mystifying, and confusing tangles and webs to be deciphered.

Not only did Laing understand individual experience and agency by using a social phenomenology that stayed close to experience, but he treated the concept of relationship in new ways. He realized that the self needs to be understood in the context of others and that experience could be of many kinds as inner, outer, and inter-experience that has its own rationale. Laing did not act in a vacuum. He was influenced by increasing interest in relationship and mutuality in psychoanalysis as expressed in the Hungarian psychoanalyst Sandor Ferenczi's work and that of the object relations schools in the UK, which included his analyst, Charles Rycroft; his clinical supervisor, D. W. Winnicott; and other Tavistock Clinic analysts, as well as the interpersonal schools.

During the early 1960s Laing moved into developing social phenomenology, going beyond existentialism of the individual and 'the other' in quite specific ways. Not only individual intentions but the context of understanding how they were perceived by others in relationships were crucial to understanding the individual. Laing followed Sartre's publications, *Search for a Method, Critique of Dialectical Reason*, and *Saint Genet*, which Laing and David Cooper summarized as *Reason and Violence* (Laing and Cooper, 1964). These works introduced seminal ideas and essential tools for situating individual choice within the context of the functioning and nature of relationships and groups. Laing adapted Sartre's philosophical concepts of praxis and process, the role of social mediations, and the way groups functioned in certain ways. In particular, Laing and Esterson adopted these ideas to researching families operating as serial and nexal groups (Laing and Esterson, 1964). Along these lines, Laing also researched interpersonal perceptions and the politics of families. Gregory Bateson's double-bind theory of schizophrenia was applied to the functioning of families. To whatever extent this theory was valid or invalid for the families of schizophrenics, it was very useful for mapping the way people interact and their consequences.

It is important to note that Laing's theories of the relationship between madness and families have in large part been greatly misinterpreted. He is often seen as being opposed to the nuclear family, which, allegedly, was the cause of pathology in individual designated members and which was supposed to stymie individuality and produce mere compliance – Laing's position has often been wrongly confused with David Cooper's position (see Cooper, 1967, 1971, 1974). Laing was falsely accused of blaming parents or the family for having created schizophrenia. This has been a widespread but fundamental misunderstanding of the nature of the research by Laing and his colleagues into families. It wasn't about trying to find the pathological source of schizophrenia, as one of Laing's colleagues at the Tavistock Clinic, John Bowlby, insisted. Laing told Bob Mullan:

> I could never get Bowlby to get the point that I wasn't trying to do a piece of research that would be decidable; the issue wasn't the decidability of whether the pathology of the patient induced the pathology of the family or whether there was family pathology. I didn't want to talk about the family pathology but you could never stop them talking about the 'family pathology'. I was interested in the communicational phenomenology that went on in the families of diagnosed schizophrenics.
>
> (Mullan, 1995, p. 274)

It was, Laing told Mullan, originally meant 'to be a study of communicationnàla Bateson rather than a study of families' (Mullan, 1995, p. 275).

Laing sharply distinguishes causation from treatment, aetiology from therapy. He told Bob Mullan:

> I'm not talking about the aetiology of schizophrenia. . . . I'm talking about the experience and behaviour that leads someone to be diagnosed as schizophrenic is more socially intelligible than has come to be supposed by most psychiatrists and most people.

He adds,

> That is a very embarrassing statement and people can't hear that, and so it means that is it translated into saying that families cause schizophrenia and therefore if you've got a schizophrenic child, you ought to feel guilty about it and that therefore there are schizophrenic associations in families, etc.
>
> (Mullan, 1995, p. 379)

Based on his data from interviews with families and his ideas about communications, Laing introduced the concepts of mystification and confusion in order to understand the modus operandi that beset many families. These can be seen as consequences of acting in dysfunctional ways.

But it is not either/or. This kind of divide can be seen in therapy: on the one hand, from the starting point of intention, experience, and interpretation, one set of events emerges. On the other hand, from the standpoint of neurological or behavioral processes, another set is described. The aims and measuring instruments are quite different. Psychoanalysis begins and ends with words and images, using the language of the lived experience of persons, separate points of view, and experiencing subjects, whereas natural scientific accounts adopt different assumptions and criteria. They both might be valid in their own terms and what they describe. There is also a distinction between clinical theory and meta-theory. It depends on the particular questions we are investigating, in recognizing and following through, staying close to the phenomena. As Laing put it in *The Divided Self*, a science is what is appropriate to its field. He was exploring the appropriate way of understanding human behavior in terms of agency and how natural scientific approaches became mixed up in this field. This was by no means an attack on natural scientific method as such, but rather the direct application where agency was involved – a confusion of praxis and process.

Laing challenged assumptions and brought existential and communications issues to therapy in a new way. In his lecture to the first conference on 'The Evolution of Psychotherapy' in Phoenix in 1985, Laing says there are 'two ways of defining what is going on –in terms of process (suffering from a mental disorder) or in terms of praxis (intentional choice-in-action)'. Laing offers two strategies in response – in terms of process, treatment of [the patient's] disorder – in terms of praxis, to treat the patient as a person. Treatment then is the way we treat the patient (Laing, 2013, p. 207). We get different results using different methodologies and criteria.

Laing argues,

> Everyone knows we are affected by our nearest and dearest. It is devilishly difficult to study the ordinariness of everyday life where most of our clients' happiness and unhappiness arise. Cartesian-Galilean natural science does not help us here, for *our* theory must be explicitly designed to *see* the world of personal passions, intentions and actions, that is, *praxis*, as well as *process*. Niels Bohr's concept of complementarity may help us here. Any cogent coherent psychotherapy must both draw on and contribute to the pragmatic knowledge, the knowledge-in-action, of how we affect each other, personally.

Laing suggests,

> the divide between fact and feelings is a product of schizoid constructions, which is not useful in the practice of psychotherapy. In reality, the reasons of the heart (praxis) and the physiology of the brain (process) coexist and are interdependent.
>
> (Laing, 2013, p. 209)

For Laing, direct, one-way causal explanations are often as simplistic as they are inaccurate. The whole system militates in certain directions, and a number of interacting biological, personal, interpersonal, historical, sociological, and cultural factors inevitably come into play. Laing was a sophisticated and complex thinker who mostly didn't reduce complex problems into black and white causes such as schizophrenia is just a social creation, psychotics are created by oppressive families, etc. He wasn't a closed system thinker and was always questioning taken-for-granted assumptions that have marred our way of understanding the most complex entities around: us all too human beings.

The 1960s were Laing's most generative period, the decade of his major contributions. I want to highlight here the significant developments revealed in Laing's important but not well-known chapter in an edited book for professionals, *Intensive Family Therapy*, in 1965. Laing meant that chapter, 'Mystification, Confusion and Conflict', to be part of a series of papers focussing on mystification and confusion and utilizing the concept of enduring interest to Laing of 'tangential communication', a form of dysfunctional communication.

The concept of mystification together with the consequences of confusion and conflict represent considerable advances in Laing's understanding of mental illness and therapy beyond *The Divided Self* in 1960 and *The Self and Others* in 1961. Laing adapts Marx's concept of 'mystification' to add the forms of reciprocal interaction of person with person to the psychological realm. Marx uses the idea of mystification to explain what happens when social relations are obscured or how far social relations form the world. The classic example is Marx's concept of the 'fetishism of commodities' – when things come to seem they have a life of their own. Laing uses Marx's model of mystification to mean, in Laing's words,

> a plausible misrepresentation of what is going on (process) or what is being done (praxis) in the service of the interests of one socioeconomic class (the exploiters) over or against another class (the exploited). By representing forms of exploitation as forms of benevolence, the exploiters bemuse the exploited into feeling at one with their exploiters, or into feeling gratitude for what (unrealized by them) in their exploitation, and, not least, into feeling bad or mad even to think of rebellion.
>
> (Laing, 1965, p. 343)

For Laing, individuals are not islands, and interactions and perceptions mould behaviour and judgment of experience. So Laing suspected that there may be different interactions within families, especially those with schizophrenics as members. His research with Aaron Esterson at the Tavistock Clinic involved 100 families and resulted in *Sanity, Madness and the Family*. Laing understood the nature of our inevitable interactions as involving communication, ascription, and commands that needed decrypting. He states:

> To mystify, in the active sense, is to befuddle, cloud, obscure, mask whatever is going on, whether this be experience, action, or process, or whatever is "the issue". It induces confusion in the sense that there is failure to see what is "really" being experienced, or being done, or going on, and failure to distinguish or discriminate the actual issues. This entails the substitution of false for true constructions of what is being experienced, being done (praxis), or going on (process), and the substitution of false issues for the actual issues. The *state* of mystification, mystification in a passive sense, is possibly, though not necessarily, a *feeling* of being muddled or confused. The act of mystification, by definition, tends to induce, if not neutralized by counteraction, a state of mystification

or confusion, not necessarily felt as such. It may or may not induce secondary conflicts, and these may or may not be recognized as such by the persons involved.

(Laing, 1965, p. 344)

For Laing, mystification takes several forms that can be dissected. It can involve confusing these modalities of feelings and states in relation to reality – such as 'you just imagined that' or 'you must have dreamt it'. Or it might involve disconfirming someone's experience and replacing it with one's own. As in

A child is playing noisily in the evening; his mother is tired and wants him to go to bed. A straight statement would be: 'I am tired. I want you to go to bed' *or* 'Go to bed, because I say so' *or* 'Go to bed because it's your bedtime'. A mystifying way to induce the child to go to bed would be: 'I'm sure you feel tired, darling, and want to go to bed now, don't you?'
  Mystification occurs here in different respects. What is ostensibly an attribution about how the child feels (you are tired) is "really" a command (go to bed). The child is told how he feels (he may or may not feel or be tired), and what he is told he feels is what mother feels herself (projective identification).

(Laing, 1965, p. 345)

Or it might be connected with rights and obligations when a person seems to have a right to determine the experience of another or someone is under an obligation to experience or not experience himself or others in a particular way.

When mystification takes place, Laing found in the families of schizophrenics that there was a significant lack in the recognition of others as their own centres of orientation. In Laing's view, 'the mystified person is operating in terms that have been misdefined for him' (Laing, 1965, p. 352). Perhaps without realizing it, the person is in an untenable position, and attempting to escape in the mystified situation may further deepen the mystifications. The practical aim of therapy is to demystify what is going on by revealing and clarifying this mapping.

Hence, we can understand what Laing terms 'the mystification of experience' in *The Politics of Experience*, where, as Laing put it,

Human beings relate to each other not simply externally, like two billiard balls, but by the relations of the two worlds of experience that come into play when two people meet. If human beings are not studied as human beings, then this . . . is violence and mystification.

(Laing, 1967, p. 53)

Laing's research on mystification and interactions led to the importance of differentiating between commands and ascriptions, somebody imputing my feelings at the same time as invalidating them as I do to myself. I think it is important not to apportion blame and victimhood here, though sometimes of course it is justified when people take advantage of others' vulnerability. I don't believe it has been shown that the double-bind theory of schizophrenia is that helpful as such. But what is helpful is respect for the person and their experience and not being dismissed as persons.

Laing defines 'diagnosis' etymologically as 'seeing through'. That is ambiguous, as it can be seen *through* to the other side, or it can be *seen* through the lens of. Part of mystification and the assumptions behind it is confusion, mis-defining, that nobody sees through. Everyone is lost without a map, beset by the consequences of not seeing what is in front of us, the obvious, although the ever-increasing complexity of the web that we weave doesn't help. The publication of *Knots* (Laing, 1970) revealed some of the forms of such knots, even if they weren't untangled. Part of Laing's increasing interest in Buddhism, I think, derived from trying to go beyond monistic systems with fixed, contradictory starting assumptions into perspectives encompassing cascading meta-contexts.

Laing develops these ideas about mystification and communications further in *The Politics of the Family* (Laing, 1971), much of which was originally delivered as the CBC Massey Lectures in 1968. There he applied the theory of sets and mapping, which were being applied to anthropology and social science, to what he termed 'the "psychosocial interior" of families in our own society' (p. 66). He discusses the mystifying mechanism of conflation of levels, the attribution of a state of affairs in a subject that is in reality a command.

> One way to get someone to *do* what one wants, is to give an order. To get someone to *be* what one wants him to be, or supposes he is or is afraid he is (whether or not this is what one wants), that is, to get him to embody one's projections, is another matter. In a hypnotic (or similar) context, one does not tell him what *to be*, but tells him what he is. Such *attributions*, in context, are many times more powerful than orders. . . . An instruction need not be defined as an instruction. It is my impression that we receive most of our earliest and most lasting instructions in the form of attributions. One is, say, told one *is* a bad boy or girl, not only instructed *to be* a good or bad boy or girl. One may be subject to both, but if one *is* (this or that), it is not necessary to be told to be what one has already been 'given to understand' one is. The key medium for communication of this kind is probably not verbal language When attributions have the function of instructions or injunctions, this function may be denied, giving rise to one type of *mystification*, akin to, or identical with, hypnotic suggestion. Hypnosis may be an experimental model of a naturally occurring phenomenon in many families.
>
> (pp. 78–79)

Laing suggests,

> I consider many adults (including myself) are, or have been, in a hypnotic trance, induced in early infancy: we remain in this state until –when we dead awaken as Ibsen makes one of his characters say – we shall find that we have never lived.

Attempts to wake before our time are often punished, especially by those who love us most. Because they, bless them, are asleep. They think anyone who wakes up, or who, still asleep, realizes that what it takes to be real is a 'dream' is going crazy. Anyone in this transitional state is likely to be confused. To indicate this confusion is a sign of illness, is a quick way to create psychosis.

(Laing, 1971, p. 82)

Notwithstanding the hyperbole of the 1960s, this conveys an important point. Therapy involves demystification, perhaps, like hypnosis, revealing instructions or suggestions that we don't realize we are carrying out and are not aware that we have even experienced. This means tracing and dissolving the suggestion involved in the mystification, which means getting to the root of the suggestion and perhaps finding a counter-suggestion or, if you like, a counter-narrative, to replace it. I wonder whether some of the intransigence and attraction in the radicalization of ISISoperatives, for example, has such a basis in a form of hypnotic suggestion. ISIS videos evince a trance-like quality, which, I think, involves a large amount of hypnotic suggestion. A successful deradicalization program, might trace suggestions back to their sources and offer alternative counter-suggestions and counter-narratives to cancel them. The therapy involves demystification as a form of debriefing and re-entry. In his fascinating paper, "A Psychoanalyst Looks at a Hypnotist', Albert Mason suggests that 'hypnotism is a folie a deux caused by mutual projective identification between two people and that in a less dramatic form this condition commonly occurs in normal development as well as in pathological psychological states' (Mason, 1994, p. 641). He cites several cases to illustrate these ideas.

In Laing's unpublished lecture 'Psychotherapy and Meditation' at the Roundhouse in London on June 26, 1977, he focused on psychotherapy and the extraordinary power of words. Speaking of the difficulty of establishing the truth value of constructions and interpretations, Laing proposes that psychotherapy consists of examining such problematic matters together. He declares:

A lot of people tend to disparage psychotherapy because they say it's simply words, which I think is an extraordinary thing to say, because you might say the splitting that besets a lot of us, psychotherapists as well as patients, often takes the form of a dissociation of feeling and realization, what one might call realization from words. Nevertheless, that doesn't decide the reality of human speech and human attributes which in the verbal form has got a capacity second to none I think for affecting us all; affecting us profoundly and immediately in our vegetative system and through all our bioenergetics system and immediately resonated by the right word or the wrong word.

Laing makes a telling point:

And I don't know any single agency that is as powerful as words. And it's just this dissociation of words, and of real speech into what Heidegger and other people have called mere talk and chatter, and babble, etc. that is one of the forms of dissociation which psychotherapy is especially set up to facilitate mending. I think one consistently recurring reason for this in my experience is the way words have been experienced by so many of us as inducing confusion or irreconcilable conflict, by setting up injunctions against the flow of natural life process.

Laing suggests that those entangled in such ways can be helped greatly by working with a psychotherapist who understands these dimensions. It's hard to do it oneself given an overriding injunction not to see what is going on, especially if one is 'caught in that spell'. He recalls his earlier proposition that this 'is not merely analogous but homologous with hypnosis, and that a number of us from our early childhood may have fallen into a hypnotic state that is lifelong'. He sees hypnosis as 'an experimental reproduction of a state which is endemic and occurs with a certain frequency in our world'.

These powerful ideas help us understand the major impact of the interaction of different levels and forms of words, situating them within their surrounding contexts and meta-contexts in the interactions of persons and groups. Words are not just tools to an end. The untangling of knots, revealing confusions and distortions, clarifying different, often conflicting, levels of communications, in general demystification of the halls of mirrors and mazes we find ourselves in, are crucial tasks for therapy. We might revisit how Breuer and Freud began with hypnosis but became side-tracked into focusing on the content of what was revealed instead of understanding the process through which it was revealed.

In lectures delivered in London in 1976 about Freud's *Introductory Lectures on Psychoanalysis* (Laing, 1976), Laing found himself very much in tune with Freud's depiction of neurosis as a conflict between two *levels* of conscious and unconscious wishes. In 1917, Freud demonstrated a clear understanding of the importance of levels. Freud stated,

> The pathogenic conflict in neurotics is not to be confused with a normal struggle between mental impulses both of which are on the same psychological footing. In the former case the dissension is between two powers, one of which has made its way to the stage of what is preconscious or conscious while the other has been held back at the stage of the unconscious. For that reason the conflict cannot be brought to an issue; the disputants can no more come to grips than, in the familiar simile, a polar bear and a whale. A true decision can only be reached when they both meet on the same ground. To make this possible is, I think, the sole task of our therapy.
>
> (Freud, 1916–17[1963], p. 433)

In an important sense, the neurotic is *mystified* by the symptoms on different levels, including levels of fantasy and reality. In my view, Laing was able to continue Freud's demystifying therapeutic journey in revealing still more levels and modalities of the struggles and confusions between different actions and desires, unmasking discrete levels of communication and miscommunication between persons such that people are better able to recognize their desires and act in alignment with them.

References

Cooper, D. (1967). *Psychiatry and anti-psychiatry*. London: Tavistock.

Cooper, D. (1971). *The death of the family*. London: Allen Lane, The Penguin Books.

Cooper, D. (1974). *The grammar of living*. New York: Pantheon.

Freud, S. (1916–17[1963]). Introductory lectures on psycho-analysis, Part 3. In J. Strachey (ed. and Trans.), *The standard edition of the complete psychological works of Sigmund Freud*, Vol. 16. London: Hogarth.

Laing, R. D. (1965). Mystification, confusion and conflict. In I. Boszormenyi-Nagy and J. L. Framozz (eds.), *Intensive family therapy*, pp. 343–363. New York: Harper and Row.

Laing, R. D. (1967). *The politics of experience and the bird of paradise*. Harmondsworrth: Penguin Books.

Laing, R. D. (1970). *Knots*. New York: Pantheon.

Laing, R. D. (1971). *The politics of the family and other essays*. London: Tavistock.

Laing, R. D. (1976). *Freud's introductory lectures*. Part 1, June 13; Part 2, July 4. London. Unpublished transcript.

Laing, R. D. (1977). Psychotherapy and meditation. *Lecture delivered at the Roundhouse London*, June 26. Unpublished transcript.

Laing, R. D. (2013). The use of existential phenomenology in psychotherapy. In J. Zeig (ed.), *The evolution of psychotherapy*, pp. 203–210. New York: Routledge.

Laing, R. D. and Cooper, D. G. (1964). *Reason and violence: A decade of Sartre's philosophy*. London: Tavistock.

Laing, R. D. and Esterson, A. (1964). *Sanity, madness and the family: Families of schizophrenics*. Harmondsworth: Penguin Books.

Mason, A. (1994). A psychoanalyst looks at a hypnotist. *Psychoanalytic Quarterly*, LXIII: 641–679.

Mullan, R. (1995). *Mad to be normal: Conversations with R. D. Laing*. London: Free Association Books.

Chapter 6

Science and Spirituality

Fritjof Capra, PhD

Spirit and Spirituality

To begin this discussion, it is useful to review the original meaning of "spirit." The Latin *spiritus* means "breath," and this is also true for the related Latin word *anima*, the Greek *psyche*, and the Sanskrit *atman*. The common meaning of these key terms indicates that the original meaning of spirit in many ancient philosophical and religious traditions, in the West as well as in the East, is that of the breath of life. Spirit – the breath of life – is what we have in common with all living beings. It nourishes us and keeps us alive.

Spirituality is usually understood as a way of being that flows from a certain profound experience of reality, which is known as a "mystical," "religious," or "spiritual" experience. There are numerous descriptions of this experience in the literature of the world's religions, which tend to agree that it is a direct, non-intellectual experience of reality with some fundamental characteristics that are independent of cultural and historical contexts.

One of the most beautiful contemporary descriptions can be found in a short essay titled "Spirituality as Common Sense," by the Benedictine monk, psychologist, and author David Steindl-Rast (1990). In accordance with the original meaning of spirit as the breath of life, Brother David characterizes spiritual experience as moments of heightened aliveness. Our spiritual moments are those moments when we feel most intensely alive. The aliveness felt during such a "peak experience," as psychologist Abraham Maslow called it, involves not only the body but also the mind.

Buddhists refer to this heightened mental alertness as "mindfulness," and they emphasize that mindfulness is deeply rooted in the body. Spirituality, then, is always embodied. Spiritual experience is an experience of aliveness of mind and body as a unity. Moreover, this experience of unity transcends not only the separation of mind and body but also the separation of self and world. The central awareness in these spiritual moments is a profound sense of oneness with all, a sense of belonging to the universe a whole.

This sense of oneness with the natural world is fully borne out by the new systemic conception of life (see Capra and Luisi, 2014). As we understand how

DOI: 10.4324/9781003564294-8

the roots of life reach deep into basic physics and chemistry, how the unfolding of complexity began long before the formation of the first living cells, and how life has evolved for billions of years by using again and again the same basic patterns and processes, we realize how tightly we are connected with the entire fabric of life.

Spirituality and Religion

When we discuss the relationship between science and spirituality, it is important to distinguish between spirituality and religion. Spirituality is a way of being grounded in a certain experience of reality that is independent of cultural and historical contexts. Religion is the organized attempt to understand spiritual experience, to interpret it with words and concepts, and to use this interpretation as the source of moral guidelines for the religious community.

There are three basic aspects to religion: theology, morals, and ritual (see Capra and Steindl-Rast, 1991, p. 12ff.). In theistic religions, theology is the intellectual interpretation of the spiritual experience, of the sense of belonging, with God as the ultimate reference point. Morals, or ethics, are the rules of conduct derived from that sense of belonging, and ritual is the celebration of belonging by the religious community. All three of these aspects – theology, morals, and ritual – depend on the religious community's historical and cultural contexts.

Theology

Theology was originally understood as the intellectual interpretation of the theologians' own mystical experience. Indeed, during the first thousand years of Christianity, virtually all of the leading theologians – the so-called "Church Fathers" – were also mystics. Over the subsequent centuries, however, during the scholastic period, theology became progressively fragmented and divorced from the spiritual experience that was originally at its core.

With the new emphasis on purely intellectual theological knowledge came a hardening of the language. Whereas the Church Fathers repeatedly asserted that religious experience cannot be adequately expressed in words, and therefore expressed their interpretations in terms of symbols and metaphors, the scholastic theologians formulated the Christian teachings in dogmatic language and required the faithful to accept these formulations as the literal truth. In other words, Christian theology became more and more rigid and fundamentalist, devoid of authentic spirituality.

The awareness of these subtle relationships between religion and spirituality is important when we compare both of them with science. While scientists try to explain natural phenomena, the purpose of a spiritual discipline is not to provide a description of the world. Its purpose, rather, is to facilitate experiences that will change a person's self and way of life. However, in the interpretations of their experiences mystics and spiritual teachers are often led to also make statements about the nature of reality, the nature of human consciousness, and the like. This allows us to compare their descriptions of reality with corresponding descriptions by scientists.

In these spiritual traditions – for example, in the various schools of Buddhism – the mystical experience is always primary; its descriptions and interpretations are considered secondary and tentative, insufficient to fully describe the spiritual experience. In a way, these descriptions are not unlike the limited and approximate models in science, which are always subject to further modifications and improvements.

In the history of Christianity, by contrast, theological statements about the nature of the world or about human nature were often considered literal truths, and any attempt to question or modify them was deemed heretical. This rigid position of the Church led to the well-known conflicts between science and fundamentalist Christianity, which have continued to the present day.

A Sense of Awe

Spiritual experience – the direct, non-intellectual experience of reality in moments of heightened aliveness – is known as a mystical experience because it is an encounter with mystery. Spiritual teachers throughout the ages have insisted that the experience of a profound sense of connectedness, of belonging to the cosmos as a whole, which is the central characteristic of mystical experience, is ineffable – that is, incapable of being adequately expressed in words or concepts – and they often describe it as being accompanied by a deep sense of awe and wonder together with a feeling of great humility.

Scientists, in their systematic observations of natural phenomena, do not consider their experience of reality as ineffable. On the contrary, we attempt to express it in technical language, including mathematics, as precisely as possible. However, the fundamental interconnectedness of all phenomena is a dominant theme also in modern science, and many of our great scientists have expressed their sense of awe and wonder when faced with the mystery that lies beyond the limits of their theories. Albert Einstein, for one, repeatedly expressed these feelings, as in the following celebrated passage (quoted in Schilpp, 1949, p. 5):

> The fairest thing we can experience is the mysterious. It is the fundamental emotion which stands at the cradle of true art and true science . . . the mystery of the eternity of life, and the inkling of the marvelous structure of reality, together with the single-hearted endeavor to comprehend a portion, be it ever so tiny.

The Divine

In theistic religions, the sense of mystery that is at the core of spiritual experience is associated with the divine. Thus, in the Christian tradition, the encounter with

mystery is an encounter with God, and the Christian mystics repeatedly emphasized that the experience of God transcends all words and concepts. Thus, Diony-
sius the Areopagite, a highly influential mystic of the early sixth century, writes:
"At the end of all our knowing, we shall know God as the unknown," and Saint
John of Damascus in the early eighth century wrote: "God is above all knowing
and above all essence."

However, most Christian theologians do want to speak about their experience
of God, and to do so, the Church Fathers used poetic language, symbols, and metaphors. The central error of fundamentalist theologians in subsequent centuries
was, and is, to adopt a literal interpretation of these religious metaphors. Once
this is done, any dialogue between religion and science becomes frustrating and
unproductive.

Ethics, Ritual, and the Sacred

Morals, or ethics, are the rules of conduct derived from the sense of belonging
that lies at the core of the spiritual experience, and ritual is the celebration of that
belonging. Both ethics and ritual develop within the context of a spiritual, or religious, community. Ethical behavior is always related to the particular community
to which we belong. When we belong to a community, we behave accordingly. In
today's world, there are two relevant communities to which we all belong. We are
all members of humanity, and we all belong to the global biosphere. We are members of *oikos*, the Earth Household, which is the Greek root of the word "ecology,"
and as such we should behave as the other members of the household behave – the
plants, animals, and microorganisms that form the vast network of relationships
that we call the web of life.

The outstanding characteristic of the Earth Household is its inherent ability to
sustain life. As members of the global community of living beings, it behooves us
to behave in such a way that we do not interfere with this inherent ability. This is
the essential meaning of ecological sustainability.

As members of the human community, our behavior should reflect a respect of
human dignity and basic human rights. Since human life encompasses biological,
cognitive, and social dimensions, human rights should be respected in all three of
these dimensions.

To lay this out in detail is quite a challenge, but fortunately we have a magnifi-
cent document that covers the broad range of human dignity and human rights. It
is called the Earth Charter (see Rockefeller, 2015). It is a global declaration of 16
values and principles for building a just, sustainable, and peaceful world – a perfect
summary of the ethics we need for our time.

Finally, returning to the three aspects of religion, there is ritual. The original
purpose of religious communities was to provide opportunities for their members
to relive the mystical experiences of the religion's founders. For this purpose, religious leaders designed special rituals within their historical and cultural contexts.

These rituals may involve special places, robes, music, psychedelic drugs, and various ritualistic objects. In many religions, these special means to facilitate mystical experience become closely associated with the religion itself and are considered sacred.

Modern Physics and Eastern Mysticism

I have now established the proper framework for talking about science and spirituality. As I have mentioned, scientists and spiritual teachers pursue very different goals. While the purpose of the former is to find explanations of natural phenomena, that of the latter is to change a person's self and way of life. However, in their different pursuits, both are led to make statements about the nature of reality that can be compared.

Among the first modern scientists to make such comparisons were some of the leading physicists of the twentieth century who had struggled to understand the strange and unexpected reality revealed to them in their explorations of atomic and subatomic phenomena. In the 1950s, several of these scientists published popular books about the history and philosophy of quantum physics, in which they hinted at remarkable parallels between the worldview implied by modern physics and the views of Eastern spiritual and philosophical traditions.

During the 1960s, there was a strong interest in Eastern spiritual traditions in Europe and North America, and many scholarly books on Hinduism, Buddhism, and Taoism were published by Eastern and Western authors. At that time, the parallels between these Eastern traditions and modern physics were discussed more frequently, and a few years later I explored them systematically in my first book *The Tao of Physics* (Capra, 1975).

My main thesis in this book is that the approaches of physicists and mystics, even though they seem at first quite different, share some important characteristics. To begin with, their method is thoroughly empirical. Physicists derive their knowledge from experiments; mystics from meditative insights. Both are observations, and in both fields these observations are acknowledged as the only source of knowledge. The objects of observation are, of course, very different in the two cases. The mystic looks within and explores his consciousness at various levels, including the physical phenomena associated with the mind's embodiment.

The physicist, by contrast, begins his inquiry into the essential nature of things by studying the material world. Exploring ever deeper realms of matter, he becomes aware of the essential unity of all natural phenomena. More than that, he also realizes that he himself and his consciousness are an integral part of this unity. Thus the mystic and the physicist arrive at the same conclusion; one starting from the inner realm, the other from the outer world. The harmony between their views confirms the ancient Indian wisdom that *brahman*, the ultimate reality without, is identical to *atman*, the reality within.

A further important similarity between the ways of the physicist and the mystic is the fact that their observations take place in realms that are inaccessible to the ordinary senses. In modern physics, these are the realms of the atomic and subatomic world; in mysticism, they are non-ordinary states of consciousness in which the everyday sensory world is transcended. In both cases, access to these non-ordinary levels of experience is possible only after long years of training within a rigorous discipline, and in both fields the "experts" assert that their observations often defy expressions in ordinary language.

After the publication of *The Tao of Physics* in 1975, numerous books appeared in which physicists and other scientists presented similar explorations of the parallels between physics and mysticism. Other authors extended their inquiries beyond physics, finding similarities between Eastern thought and certain ideas about free will; death and birth; and the nature of life, mind, consciousness, and evolution. Moreover, the same kinds of parallels have been drawn also to Western mystical traditions.

Some of these explorations were initiated by Eastern spiritual teachers. The Dalai Lama, in particular, hosted a series of dialogues with Western scientists on "Mind & Life" at his home in Dharamsala.

Deep Ecology and Spirituality

The extensive explorations of the relationships between science and spirituality over the past three decades have made it evident that the sense of oneness, which is the key characteristic of spiritual experience, is fully confirmed by the understanding of reality in contemporary science. Hence, there are numerous similarities between the worldviews of mystics and spiritual teachers – both Eastern and Western – and the systemic conception of nature that is now being developed in several scientific disciplines.

The awareness of being connected with all of nature is particularly strong in ecology. Connectedness, relationship, and interdependence are fundamental concepts of ecology, and connectedness, relationship, and belonging are also the essence of religious experience. I believe therefore that ecology – and in particular the philosophical school of deep ecology, is the ideal bridge between science and spirituality.

When we look at the world around us, we find that we are not thrown into chaos and randomness but are part of a great order, a grand symphony of life. Every molecule in our body was once a part of previous bodies – living or non-living – and will be a part of future bodies. In this sense, our body will not die but will live on, again and again, because life lives on. Moreover, we share not only life's molecules but also its basic principles of organization with the rest of the living world. Indeed, we belong to the universe, and this experience of belonging can make our lives profoundly meaningful.

References

Capra, F. (1975). *The Tao of physics*. Boulder, CO: Shambhala.

Capra, F. and Luisi, P. L. (2014). *The systems view of life*. New York: Cambridge University Press.

Capra, F. and Steindl-Rast, D. (1991). *Belonging to the universe*. San Francisco: Harper.

Rockefeller, S. (2015). *Democratic equality, economic equality, and the earth charter*. Earth Charter International.

Schilpp, P. A. (ed.) (1949). *Albert Einstein: Philosopher-scientist*. Evanston, IL: Library of Living Philosophers.

Steindl-Rast, D. (1990). Spirituality as common sense. *The Quest*, 3, no. 2.

III

What Are Altered States?

Chapter 7

The Nature of Reality

Some Personal Reflections

Fritjof Capra, PhD

Traditionally, questions about the essential nature of reality are asked by philosophers. At the dawn of Western philosophy, in ancient Greece, Thales declared that "all things are full of gods." For Heraclitus, the universal principle was fire, a symbol for the continuous flows and changes in the material world. Pythagoras taught that the essential nature of things lies in number, or "pattern," as we would say today.

At the same time, the Indian sages declared that there is no objective reality, independent of our measuring and categorizing mind. To think that the shapes and structures around us are objective realities of nature is *maya*, an illusion, in their view.

Quantum Physics

In the twentieth century, questions about the essential nature of reality were asked for the first time by scientists as well. During the first three decades of the century, the exploration of the atomic and subatomic world brought physicists in contact with a strange and unexpected reality that shattered the foundations of their worldview and forced them to think in entirely new ways.

Nothing like that had ever happened in science. Revolutions like those of Copernicus and Darwin had introduced profound changes in the general conception of the universe, changes that were shocking to many people, but the new concepts themselves were not difficult to grasp. In the twentieth century, however, the quantum physicists faced a serious challenge to their ability to understand the universe. Every time they asked nature a question in an atomic experiment, nature answered with a paradox, and the more they tried to clarify the situation, the sharper the paradoxes became.

In their struggle to grasp this new reality, scientists became painfully aware that their basic concepts, their language, and their whole way of thinking were inadequate to describe atomic phenomena. Their problem was not only intellectual but involved an intense emotional and even existential crisis as well.

Their struggle was vividly described by Werner Heisenberg in his classic account *Physics and Philosophy* (Heisenberg, 1958). The book is a scholarly work, quite technical at times, but also full of personal, and even highly emotional, passages.

DOI: 10.4324/9781003564294-10

I read Heisenberg's book as a young student in Austria, and at the age of nineteen I did not by any means understand all of it. In fact, most of it remained a mystery for me at this first reading, but it sparked a fascination with that epochal period of science that has never left me.

Heisenberg's book remained my companion during my student years and beyond. Looking back on this time, I can see that it was Heisenberg who planted the seed that would mature, more than a decade later, in my systematic investigation of the limits of the Cartesian worldview. "The Cartesian partition," wrote Heisenberg (meaning the separation of mind and matter), "has penetrated deeply into the human mind during the three centuries following Descartes, and it will take a long time for it to be replaced by a really different attitude toward the problem of reality" (Heisenberg, 1958, p. 81). Quantum physics showed scientists "a new reality," and from that time on, the nature of reality became a popular subject of discussion not only in philosophy but also in science.

The Sixties

Between my student years in Vienna and the writing of my first book, *The Tao of Physics* (Capra, 1975), lies the period of my life during which I experienced the most profound and most radical personal transformation: the period of the 1960s. For those of us who identify with the cultural movements of "the sixties," this period represents not so much a decade as a state of mind, characterized by an expansion of consciousness, a radical questioning of authority in a wide variety of fields, a sense of empowerment, and the experience of sensuous beauty and community.

During the 1960s, I began to study Eastern mysticism. I experimented with psychedelic drugs, and I began to practice meditation. All these practices involved an expansion of consciousness toward experiences involving nonordinary modes of awareness, which are traditionally achieved through meditation but may also occur in various other contexts and which psychologists at the time began to call "transpersonal." Psychedelic drugs played a significant role in that movement, as did the human potential movement's promotion of expanded sensory awareness, expressed in its exhortation, "Get out of your head and into your senses!"

A particular type of psychedelic experience were the ones described by Carlos Castaneda within the context of shamanism. Casteneda's books were immensely popular during the sixties and had a big impact on me. His second book, characteristically, was titled *A Separate Reality* (Castaneda, 1971).

The arts of the 1960s – music, film, literature, theater – also explored these altered realities by re-creating some kinds of psychedelic experiences. Examples would be the Beatles' *Sgt. Pepper* album, the free jazz of John Coltrane, the magical realism of Latin American writers like Gabriel García Márquez, the performances of the Living Theater, or the films of Fellini, Buñuel, and many others.

The expansion of consciousness we pursued in the sixties was a movement beyond materialism and toward a new spirituality, beyond ordinary reality through meditative and psychedelic experiences, and beyond rationality through expanded sensory awareness. The combined effect was a continual sense of magic, awe, and wonder that for many of us will forever be associated with the sixties.

The Tao of Physics

While I experienced these altered states of consciousness through art, psychedelics, and meditation, the "new reality" of quantum physics was always on my mind as I continued my day job as a theoretical physicist. And then, in the 1970s, I finally put the two together in a systematic exploration of the parallels between modern physics and Eastern mysticism – first in a series of articles and then in my first book, *The Tao of Physics* (Capra, 1975).

The basic thesis of *The Tao of Physics* is that the approaches of physicists and mystics, even though they seem at first quite different, share some important characteristics. To begin with, their method is thoroughly empirical. Physicists derive their knowledge from experiments; mystics from meditative insights. Both are observations, and in both fields these observations are acknowledged as the only source of knowledge.

The objects of observation are of course very different in the two cases. Mystics look within and explore their consciousness at various levels, including the physical phenomena associated with the mind's embodiment. Physicists, by contrast, begin their inquiry into the essential nature of things by studying the material world. Exploring ever deeper realms of matter, they become aware of the essential unity of all natural phenomena. More than that, they also realize that they themselves and their consciousness are an integral part of this unity. Thus the mystic and the physicist arrive at the same conclusion; one starting from the inner realm, the other from the outer world. The harmony between their views confirms the ancient Indian wisdom that *brahman*, the ultimate reality without, is identical to *atman*, the reality within.

A further important similarity between the ways of the physicist and the mystic is the fact that their observations involve experiences of "altered realities" beyond the realm of everyday sensory experience. For the physicist, it is the reality of atomic and subatomic phenomena; for the mystic, it is the reality of nonordinary states of consciousness. In both cases, access to these nonordinary levels of experience is possible only after long years of training within a rigorous discipline, and in both fields the "experts" assert that their observations often defy expressions in ordinary language. In *The Tao of Physics* I explored the similarities between those two "altered realities."

Modern Cognitive Science

In the 1970s and 1980s, cognitive scientists took another radical step in the scientific conception of the nature of reality within the context of a new systemic understanding of life. They asserted that the features of our ordinary, everyday reality, which we perceive and agree upon, are not features of an independently existing world, but are created in the very process of perception.

According to the so-called Santiago theory of cognition by Humberto Maturana and Francisco Varela (Maturana and Varela, 1987), cognition (the process of knowing) is not a representation of an independently existing world. The idea that there is an objective reality and that the living organism somehow takes a picture or produces some other representation of it in the brain is incorrect. According to the Santiago theory, cognition is a continuous process of "bringing forth," or "enacting," a world through the process of living.

In a way this generalizes the influence of the act of perception on the perceived object, which was famously analyzed in quantum physics by Werner Heisenberg, to everyday perception. And it also echoes the Hindu concept of *maya* – the idea that all forms we perceive are relative, fluid, and ever changing. Interestingly, the original meaning of *maya*, one of the most important terms in Indian philosophy, is "magic creative power."

As an example of how we bring forth a world, let us consider a tree. We look at a tree, and we see a certain outline; we see leaves, we see a trunk. Now imagine a bee – suppose it's a flowering tree – looking at the tree, or not even looking, but sensing the tree somehow. A bee with a very limited brain and nervous system will have a very different impression of the tree. So, for the bee the tree has a very different shape. Now, suppose a dog or a deer perceives the tree. Again, a very different shape.

And even in the human realm we can look at a tree when we are in a certain mood, say, when we're sort of bored and don't quite know what to do. Well, it's just a tree; it's just standing there, nothing special. Or we can be in a very euphoric mood: this is a beautiful tree; look at the light behind it! We see it differently; it's a different tree. Or you can drink a couple of whiskies and get a little drunk: the tree changes. You take some LSD – much more extreme – and suddenly the tree is flaming! So, which is the real tree?

According to the Santiago theory, there is no objectively existing tree. This does not mean that nothing exists out there. There is an existing world, but the way we divide this world into patterns and define objects like a tree depend on the way we perceive it. This is why Maturana and Varela say, "we bring forth a world" (Maturana and Varela, 1987, p. 9) in the act of perception, in the act of cognition, which, ultimately, is the act of living.

Thus, living beings with different sensory perceptions – different species or people in different states of consciousness – bring forth "different worlds" or "different realities." In other words, even our everyday reality is just one of many alternate realities.

References

Capra, F. (1975). *The Tao of physics*. Boulder, CO: Shambhala.
Castaneda, C. (1971). *A separate reality*. New York: Simon and Schuster.
Heisenberg, W. (1958). *Physics and philosophy*. New York: Harper Torchbooks.
Maturana, H. and Varela, F. (1987). *The tree of knowledge*. Boston: Shambhala.

Chapter 8

Falling in Love as an Altered State

M. Guy Thompson, PhD

What does it mean to fall in love? Can anyone fall in love, or are some people incapable of it? What exactly has to happen *in order* to fall in love? What is this phenomenon that distinguishes the notion of "falling" from other kinds of loving, even those that are sexual in nature?

The first thing we need to consider is that the word "love" is imprecise. It can mean a lot of different modes of feeling in a variety of relationships, and it may not even connote a feeling at all. Is the love a mother feels for her child, for example, the same as a young man feels for his first motorcycle? Is the love of God the same as the love for a sexual partner or the love of food? Is the love for oneself the same as the love for sunsets or the cinema? And what about the drug experience? Don't drugs elicit feelings that we associate with intense and unremitting pleasure or equanimity? Don't we sometimes take drugs to approximate the feeling of love that is missing in our lives? Clearly all these experiences are not the same, and the feelings we associate with them, even if we say we "love" every one of them, are distinct.

Falling in Love

What we call "falling in love" is first and foremost a *sexual* experience, compounded by an intense emotional connection with the person in question. There are other, non-sexualized ways of loving, but none of those occasion ***falling in love***. Enjoying sex with someone, however, in and of itself, isn't necessarily a catalyst for falling in love with that person. Great sex is pleasurable to be sure, but not necessarily complemented by a feeling of love. Love and sex aren't synonymous, but they enjoy a privileged, if mysterious, relationship. The minimum requirement for falling in love is the ***integration*** of physical, sexual attraction and a profound, loving connection with another person.

So what are the signs that you are falling in love? Say you meet a person you're attracted to, you spend an evening together and feel this amazing connection to that person. One thing leads to another and you spend the night together making love. You feel this is the most wonderful sexual experience you have ever had and you don't want the night to end. The first sign that you're falling in love is that

DOI: 10.4324/9781003564294-11

you cannot bear being separated from this person. This turns out to be an essential prerequisite for knowing that you're in love. **Love seeks *proximity*** and demands it. You want to be with this person *all the time*. You cannot bear being separated, and when you are, you think about this person constantly.

Another sign that you're falling in love is that you become ***obsessed*** with this person. You can't get them out of your mind. This is a mental way of achieving proximity when you're separated. Proximity and obsession feed on each other. This is the second sign that you're in love. Yet a third sign that you're falling for someone is an extraordinary feeling of *happiness*. If you never felt happy before, you feel it now. Your life is completely different, and everything has changed. Whatever problems you were struggling with, whether financial, your living situation, a terrible job or graduate school you feel trapped in, *doesn't matter*. You are happy, and all because this person has come into your life. You not only want to be close to this person, to touch them, kiss them, caress and hold them. You want to **be** with them, *forever*. (See Santas, 1988, for more on Plato's conception of love.) That is the fourth sign that you're in love: **you want this love to last**. This is how Plato defined love more than two thousand years ago: *love is a desire that you want to preserve in perpetuity*. Otherwise, you're just as happy to go on to the next person, and the one after that, and so on, which is what people who cannot fall in love do. After all, variety is the spice of life, isn't it? Well, when you're in love, variety is **not** the spice of life. Variety is out; perpetuity is in. Isn't this why we invented marriage? To hang onto this person for dear life?

Maybe you have felt this way for someone, and maybe you haven't. But let's say that you have. What if this person you are so in love with isn't in love with you? Or what if that person falls out of love with you and ends the relationship while you're still in love with them? How do you feel about that? Compassionate? Indifferent? Amused? Not on your life! You feel like you've just fallen off a cliff. You want to die. This is when you're thinking, "Thank God for drugs!" But drugs don't really help all that much. After all, we're talking about unrequited love, the experience that Sigmund Freud said is the most painful feeling there is. In other words, rejection sucks, and none of us take it so well. Now your life has no meaning and you can't understand how such a thing could have happened, even if you saw it coming, as we often do. And you thought you were obsessed with this person when you were in love with each other? Now you really know what it's like to be obsessed with someone, night and day, every day, without respite. And how long are we capable of being obsessed with a person who rejected us? **Some people never get over it**. They've been stuck in it all their lives and can't find a way out.

And then there's the question of judgment. Everyone knows that goes out the window the moment you fall in love. Ordinarily, we exercise at least a modicum of judgment when weighing the virtues of another person. What kind of person, for example, would you enter into a business relationship with? Or loan money to? Or embrace as a confidante, or a mentor that you trust with your life? Falling in love? All such sentiments go out the window as you impulsively put yourself at the mercy of a person who, for all you know, would just as soon cut off your head and eat you for breakfast. Judgment and love are incompatible. Yet we would put our lives on the line for such a person. Yes, you probably have to be mad to fall in love. But what kind of madness are we talking about? Is it the kind we should avoid, or a madness we should pursue because it epitomizes the best that life has to offer?

These are only some of the questions that I want to explore. I'll begin with a quote from Janet Malcolm, the psychoanalytic author and critic:

> [According to Freud, our personal relationships] are a messy tangle of *misapprehensions*, at best an *uneasy truce* between powerful solitary fantasy systems. Even romantic love is fundamentally solitary, and has at its core a profound *impersonality*. The concept of transference destroys faith in personal relations and explains why they are tragic: *we cannot know each other.*
>
> (1981, p. 6; emphasis added)

If Malcolm is correct in this dark assessment of the human condition, why is Freud's thesis – that love is an illusion – so difficult to accept? What is Freud getting at when he claims that the person I think I fell in love with isn't in fact the person I thought they were? Who, then, is this person? In order to answer this question, we first need to take a detour through the earliest stages of our childhoods, where we were first shaped, beginning with our first taste of love.

One of Freud's most original contributions to our notions about love is contained in an early book, *Three Essays on Sexuality* (1905[1953]): "The finding of an object is in fact a *refinding* of it" (p. 222). This statement is perhaps Freud's most profound contribution to our understanding of love. The child's first experience of love is at the mother's breast, or a facsimile of it, which is the most blissful experience one can imagine. It is also the prototype for all our subsequent experiences of love. That we have no memory of this experience matters not in the slightest, because it is ingrained in each of us. The connection between love and sex is also explained by this thesis, because suckling is not only a source of nourishment but a highly charged sexual experience as well – in fact, our very first. I know some of you will find this statement ludicrous. Bear with me.

Though our love for the mother and the sexual experience we enjoyed with her begins immediately after birth and persists throughout infancy, the two become split off during latency – which begins around the age of six or so. That's when the sexual portion is repressed, though its affectionate aspect survives and remains conscious. In adolescence, our sexual desires break loose from their original moorings and are directed at new, non-incestuous love objects. However, in order for this to happen, the new love must in some respects **resemble the old**, though we typically don't notice the similarities. Moreover, a second condition must be satisfied in order for this new love to blossom. Our feelings for the new person mustn't arouse the guilt that we typically associate with the original love object. Otherwise our unconscious guilt will prompt us to repress any such feelings for this person, and we won't be able to love them. According to Freud (1905 [1953]), "What is left over from the sexual relation to the first object helps to prepare for the choice of [a new] object and thus to restore the happiness that was lost" (p. 222). This implies that the experiences of love and happiness are inextricably intertwined. (See Nussbaum, 1986, for a detailed exploration of happiness.)

But how can an infant be expected to fall in love when the child experiences the mother not as a separate person, but as part of itself? Besides, both boys and girls enjoy this primary relation with the *mother* or mothering figure. What about their gender differences? Is the experience the same for girls as it is for boys? In fact, this early suckling experience only introduces the child to an amazing sense of *connectedness* to another person. It doesn't, properly speaking, introduce us to *love*. Freud was convinced, however, that it does introduce us to sex.

It's only later, when we enter the oedipal period (from roughly three to five years of age), that we *consciously* fall in love with one or both parents. Unlike the suckling experience, which is preverbal, we are acutely conscious of falling in love with this or that parental figure. But again, we repress this experience later. Freud believed that we're born bisexual so that during the oedipal phase we alternate between *both* parents, loving each in turn while experiencing the other as rival, eventually settling on one. (This would hold true even if our parents are gay.) At this point, our sexual orientation, whether gay or straight, is fixed, though we may not know it at the time. This is usually the mother for the boy and the father for the girl, but it might just as well be the opposite, and often is. Whichever the case may be, *this* is the prototype for the relationship that we seek to "refind" in another person when we reach sexual maturity at puberty. Whereas the earlier suckling experience serves as the prototype for sexual *pleasure* and the feeling of *connectedness* it engenders, it's only later during the oedipal phase that our experience of love becomes truly ***personal***. This is when we genuinely fall in love for the first time, and the parent or other close relation with whom we fall in love becomes the prototype for anyone we subsequently fall in love with as adults. The two experiences – suckling and falling in love – are comingled into a unitary experience of sexual bliss. This explains why oral sex, whether kissing, fellatio, or cunnilingus, are ways we typically recapitulate the bliss from the oral stage of development. That some people don't enjoy kissing or oral sex says something about their early nurturing experience.

Neurotic Love

Naturally, there is much in this model that can go wrong; otherwise, there would be no neuroses and, according to Freud, no psychopathology. So what does this constellation of events tell us about **neurotic** love, and how do we distinguish it from normal, happy love? *Basically, mature love is the restoration of a happiness that was lost* in early childhood. This may explain why people who fall in love often have the feeling that they've known this person forever, though they only just met. If our attachment to the parental love object was too strong, it inhibits the choice of a new love object. It's as though no one else can take their place. On the other hand, if the attachment was more subdued, resulting in greater psychic freedom, the adolescent will be able to find, and fall in love with, a new love object. Happy love is free from the ambivalence or inhibition that we associate with neurotic conflict, a conflict between desire and guilt. Neurotic love is epitomized by the inhibition that prevents us from loving another person wholeheartedly.

The other great discovery of Freud's was his theory of narcissism. This concept is crucial for understanding why people fall in love and why some people are incapable of it or of sustaining it. Freud observed that all babies are blessed with an omnipotent state of self-sufficiency. This blissful condition, short-lived as it is, will eventually diminish. The theory of narcissism implies that we begin life with two love objects, not one: the mother as well as our self. In order to free ourselves to love others, we have to free ourselves from *both*, the incestuous as well as the narcissistic. Because Freud believed that we are born bisexual, he also believed that homosexuality is a variant of normal development. In his famous essay "On Narcissism" (1914 [1957]), Freud noted that *identification* plays a crucial role when falling in love. He believed that the future gay male baby forms an intense fixation to the mother (or some other woman) and that after leaving her behind identifies with that woman and takes *himself* as a sexual object. From this basis he then looks for a young man who resembles himself and who he then loves as his mother loved him. The gay man who falls in love, in effect, becomes his mother, and his lover becomes his former self. This kind of secondary narcissism Freud distinguished from primary narcissism, which is when we fall in love with *ourselves*.

Freud's discovery of narcissistic love ranks among his greatest discoveries. One of its most important features concerns the nature of the *ego ideal*, a crucial feature of falling in love. In the first stage of narcissistic development we fall in love with *ourselves*. In the second stage this love is transferred onto the ego ideal, the person we *aspire* to be. Traditionally, we contrast self-love, the *receiving* of love, with *actively loving* another person, but Freud introduces a third option: narcissistic love. With this alternative I fall in love with a person modeled on my love for myself. There's an inevitable tension between the love I get from others, which is narcissistic, and the love I give, which is surrendered. Freud believed if I love the other person too much I deplete my narcissism, which makes me feel unworthy of love. Those with poor self-esteem will be devastated if the love relation were to end, whereas the self-confidant person will survive to love another day once their narcissism is restored.

This means that falling in love can impoverish the self to such a degree that we feel decimated. In some cases the lover's self-esteem is restored by having his or her love reciprocated, but in other cases the love object consumes the self, to the self's detriment. Moreover, there's an inevitable tension between the self and our ego ideal. We're always trying to bridge the gap between them, because the closer together they are, which is to say, the more I approximate the person I want to be, the happier I am. The further apart, the more miserable. If they are too far apart, it may result in psychosis, when we appear to be two different people. The tension between them can be beneficial or detrimental. When beneficial, the ego ideal prompts the self toward greater achievement and is the source of ambition. If excessive, it may become the totality of one's existence, as with workaholics, or a life devoted exclusively to a religion, or a political cause. This person will never be happy, because they will always feel unworthy of love. At bottom, they hate themselves.

Now for the crucial part of our discussion: What actually happens when we fall in love? When we fall in love, our ego ideal is projected onto the other person, in the same way the child idealized the parent prior to the ego ideal's formation. This means that the lover regresses back to that period in childhood when his or her idealization of the parent was most intense. When the ego ideal is projected onto this person, the tension between the self and the ego ideal is eliminated – the same process that ensues in a manic state. *When love is reciprocated, there is no finer experience.* This is what it feels like to be madly in love with another person. Now we're at the mercy of that person, and our judgment is singularly compromised. It's as though the self is now loved by the ego ideal, though this part of the experience is unconscious. *Only the blissful feeling achieves awareness, and this is about as happy as any human being can get and is the prototype for how we conceive happiness.*

Now we can begin to understand why it isn't so easy to distinguish between what it feels like to fall in love and when we have succumbed to a manic episode. In both cases the ego and ego ideal merge, an experience of intense pleasure. Judgment is abandoned, and the sudden transformation serves as the beginning of a new relationship or initiation into a psychotic episode. Phenomenologically, it is virtually impossible to tell them apart. Anyone who falls in love and gives themselves to another person has lost his (or her) senses. There is nothing rational about this experience, which is also the most remarkable thing about falling in love: the respite it gives us from the obsessive worry and relentless strategizing that the anxieties of our day-to-day existence impose on us.

Now that we have an idea of the complexity involved in falling in love, we can begin to appreciate that it isn't so easy to know whom we are falling in love with, nor even who *I* am! After all, don't we go into therapy in order to discover who we are? If we don't even know ourselves, how in the world can we presume to know others? If love compromises our judgment, it compromises our sanity as well, for sanity relies on judgment more than anything else. Love, then, is a kind of madness. But what kind of madness is it? Is it a good madness or bad? Or both? In order to answer this question, we need to look more closely at what we mean by love and the different types of experience that we designate as "love." So far, we've only been talking about one kind of love: erotic, or sexual, love. What about those ways of loving that are not specifically erotic?

Caritas

In the English language we have only one word for love, but the Greeks had several. I'm going to touch on only three: erotic love, friendly love – which the Greeks called *philia* – and the most giving kind of love possible, sympathic love, what the

Greeks termed *agapé*, but is more familiar in its Latinized form, *caritas*, literally meaning charity. I want to focus primarily on the difference between *eros* and *caritas*, the two kinds of love that ensure genuine and lasting happiness.

The Greeks saw *eros* as the most common love and the one most readily available. As we just saw, it is essentially narcissistic. Even when we love others erotically, we are in fact loving a projected image of our selves, which is mixed up with early memories of our fathers and mothers and other people in our orbit. This might explain why it is the one form of love that the Greeks associated with madness. However, erotically induced madness can either be a good, divinely sanctioned madness or the bad, demonic variety. "Our greatest blessings," says Socrates in the *Phaedrus*, "come to us by way of madness, provided the madness is given as a divine gift" (cited in Dodds, 1951, p. 64). Even before Socrates Greek literature was replete with references to Eros's dark side, a daemon spirit who is capable of savagery, injustice, drunkenness, even madness. After all, one of eros' principal features is his ability to possess and bewitch those mortals he would destroy, those who got on the wrong side of Aphrodite. As we know, that peculiar form of madness that serial killers fall prey to is always sexual in nature. They kill what they love – and they love to kill.

And yet, *eros* is also capable of giving us joy and wonder. Whether it is the good, healthy kind of madness or its opposite, erotic love is nevertheless limited. This is due to its nature. *Eros* is hungry and insatiable, which is why it seeks proximity and wants to be with the love partner in all ways and at all times. It is possessive. It is a love rooted in desire, so *eros wants* the other, wants to both receive love and give love and rejoice in the energy it unleashes. Unlike *caritas*, *eros* cannot know the other, because "mystery" is its principal vehicle and the reason it causes us to lose judgment. If I were only capable of erotic love my life would be profoundly constricted, and I would never find genuine happiness, no matter how many times I fall in love with however many people.

Philia, or friendly love, is not erotically charged. It is epitomized by the friendships we enjoy for whom we feel no sexual charge or urgency. In fact, friends, for the most part, offer us respite from the turmoil and uncertainty that occasion sexual relationships. This is why sex and therapy don't mix. If we haven't already, we learn from our therapists other ways of loving a person that are not so possessive and narcissistic, but more giving. This is what also epitomizes friendship. Successful friendships thrive on reciprocity and don't do so well when one of the friends wants to hog all the attention. Yes, we all have our share of narcissistic friends, for narcissists are usually attractive, and maybe to others *we* are the narcissistic ones, but the friends we love the most are those who give as much as they take. This is why friendship, or *philia*, is an important step toward the most giving kind of love there is, *caritas*, or what I prefer to call sympathic love, rooted in an uncommon capacity for compassion.

When psychotherapy is successful, it teaches us something about friendship, because our therapist becomes our best friend, the one person we can confide in without fear of being judged or condemned. This is a person we can trust will not use anything we tell them against us. In fact, this is what we value most in friendships, the sense of trust and fidelity they engender. The modern marriage is essentially an integration of erotic love and friendship. Marriages were originally rooted in legally binding, religiously sanctioned contracts that were *obligatory*. They were not rooted in romantic love the way they are today. Now we expect the relationship to serve both persons equally and reciprocally, not merely contractually. If such expectations are not met, the contract is usually broken. Erotic love is rooted in passion, not reciprocity, and once the passion subsides, if the reciprocity isn't there, one of the two parties will usually find the arrangement unacceptable.

Caritas is even more selfless, more giving, and less judgmental in our regard for those whom we love. Not everyone is capable of accessing it consistently. It is the only form of loving that helps us know the other person as they are, not what we project onto them. Whereas friendships still contain an element of *eros* – a bridge, as it were, between *eros* and *caritas* – *caritas* is both passionate and selfless. In relations that engender *caritas*, I seek more than proximity and affection: I hope to know *who* this person is in all her depth and complexity. And the more I know, the more I like. That's how love works: full acceptance. According to Thomas Aquinas, the thirteenth-century theologian, *caritas* consists in knowing the other as that person *is*, in his or her *is-ness*. This entails a letting-be and leaving-be, the opposite of desiring or transgressing. Without a capacity for *caritas*, we would be incapable of sympathy: the ability to know and give way to the other's innermost being. (See Thompson, 2016, for more on the concept of sympathy. See also Chapter Four.) To be with someone sympathetically means literally to *be with* that person's experience, feeling states, and suffering, without judging them. Without *caritas*, it would be difficult to be a psychotherapist. This is why we associate *caritas* with the most giving elements of loving, including a capacity for generosity, devotion, commiseration, forgiveness, trust, and mercy. None of these qualities is erotically charged per se.

Yet when we fall in love, we fall in love erotically. As we have seen, this is based almost entirely on what we project onto the other person. This occurs via happenstance. We have no way of consciously knowing what we will project, and we can't control it. It could be a smile, a conversational inflection, a look in the eyes or other idiosyncratic facial or behavioral feature that we happen to associate with someone we adored as a child, be it our mother, father, sister, brother, nursemaid, baby sitter, family friend – you name it. What they all share in common is that we loved them in our infancy and a few years beyond. If there is an equation here, it's that the earlier the love, the more powerfully it sits in our unconscious. Yet over time, these projections are not enough to sustain a relationship, as the person we begin to know in their *is-ness* surreptitiously replaces the person we fell in love with. If we enjoy a capacity for *caritas* when we began this relationship, we are also capable of falling in love with who that person genuinely is and begin to love *that* person even more deeply than the one we initially fell in love with. In this case the surviving erotic and sympathetically charged ways of loving comingle and persist after the heady intensity of the erotic edition subsides, as it inevitably will.

But what happens if you harbor an impoverished relationship with *caritas* because you're still too neurotic, ambivalent, or narcissistic to give yourself to another person? You just may be incapable of falling in love because you're still angry with that parental figure that you continue to hold onto, a figure that no one can replace because you are still in love with him, or her, and furious with them. You project all that onto the person you ostensibly fall in love with, but the resentment you harbor leaks in and drains your projections of all the goodness they momentarily enjoyed. As those projections fall away, you begin to feel the same disappointments you harbor toward that original love object. You begin to make demands that your lover change this or that about themselves, but it isn't your partner that you're trying to change, but the ghosts of your past relationships. Naturally, those demands will prove futile. We are who we are, and we can't change that. This is why you can fall in love with a person you don't even like. In fact, you may even despise this person and want nothing more than to punish and taunt them, for all the pain you insist they cause you. Yet even this isn't likely to deter you if you are in love with this person. My love for the other doesn't depend on its being reciprocated. If it were, there would be no tragedy.

The Narcissist

Without *caritas*, love cannot endure, no matter how strong the erotic component. So why is it that some people cannot fall in love? Or when they do, they can't sustain it? This, after all, is the most chronic problem that brings people into psychotherapy. We're talking about people who are only partially capable of loving others *sympathetically*. What holds them back? It seems to me that the culprit is their narcissism. These unlucky souls love themselves ambivalently, and this means they can only love *others* ambivalently as well. They are able to give, but they're more preoccupied with taking. Freud believed that loving in the non-narcissistic fashion is experienced by some as a *depleting* of their essence, and they can't give it up. They tell themselves that when they get enough love from others, *then* they will reciprocate. But they never get enough to fill that void, because there is nothing to "fill." We are openness in our essence. We are raw and unadulterated engagement. There is no inside. It takes us awhile to learn this. Meanwhile, we assume that the thing missing in our lives is that we haven't been loved enough. We simply need more. We may devote ourselves to being lovable, attractive, and charismatic in order to procure all the love we can get from our friends, lovers, family members, even perfect strangers. We have little to give because we are trying to compensate for all the things we didn't get in our troubled histories.

Narcissism is a much-abused term and no doubt confusing because it contains both healthy and unhealthy elements. But it's worth wrestling with these complexities, because we are all narcissistic, in both senses of the term. Adolescence was a profoundly narcissistic time for us, and for the most part, we're stuck in it. What does it take to become less narcissistic and more loving, less needy and more giving? The most intractable feature of narcissism is one's *touchiness*: the proverbial narcissistic injury. All of us suffer narcissistic injuries as a matter of course. It happens every day in every way. It is unavoidable. But the person we label "narcissistic" is especially thin-skinned. It doesn't take much to rub them the wrong way. And if they feel slighted, it feels like an injustice that must be corrected. Our current President is a perfect example of this character type, but admittedly his is an extreme example. Most of us are of two minds about our narcissism. We're capable of love, but not consistently. We can be giving, but we can also be punitive and paranoid and read all kinds of motives into the reasons we feel other people let us down. Paranoia and narcissism are bedfellows. And we know that paranoia is the most resistant feature of our psychopathology to insight and reflection. Jealousy is also a problem. In fact, Freud situated the jealousy that we experience at the oedipal stage as the source of our psychopathology, especially our narcissism.

Can the narcissist find happiness? In a word, only relatively and sporadically. This is because happiness never comes from what we can get, from the abundance and security we're so convinced is attainable. Happiness only comes from what we give, from our capacity to love, in the form of *caritas*, not from *being* loved – however rewarding that experience may be. *Caritas* is an inherently selfless way of loving that Buddhists and Christians alike have always known is the only true path to the equanimity we seek. This has nothing to do with ethics or morality. You can compel yourself to behave ethically, to follow the rules, but this isn't love. You may be generous out of guilt for all the crimes you've committed in the service of your success, but this will never salve your conscience or make you happy. The happiness we seek derives from loving, loving the life that we're living, the pastimes we enjoy, the friendships we commit to, the work we find rewarding, but most of all, the people we adore. There is nothing in life more rewarding than the relationships we call friends, lovers, children, colleagues – the very people in our lives with whom we choose to share *intimacy*.

Conclusion

So where does this leave us? If enduring love is predicated on our capacity for *caritas*, then it isn't a question of simply finding the right person to be with. Erotic love requires the happenstance of finding someone who triggers that recognition of this or that trait that we unconsciously associate with an early love object. Obviously, luck plays a role in this. It is a matter of chance, for example, that the two of us meet and that our projections prove compatible. But once this happens, nothing will come of that union without a well-developed capacity for selflessness, the polar opposite of erotic, narcissistic self-interest. How can we develop this capacity, if we haven't already? The answer? *Through inner work*: psychotherapy, psychoanalysis, or whatever mode of therapy you trust. This can take a long time. Some of us may pursue spiritual practices, and others will entertain uncommon forms of therapeutic engagement. If we're lucky and determined, any one of us can achieve this goal. All it takes is overcoming the self-absorption we've been committed to all our lives. This takes courage, which you no doubt know, means *openheartedness*. How do you open your heart when it's been closed for so long? That is something each of us must ask ourselves.

References

Dodds, E. R. (1951). *The Greeks and the irrational*. Berkeley, Los Angeles, and London: University of California Press.

Freud, S. (1953–1973). *The standard edition of the complete psychological works of Sigmund Freud*, Vol. 24 (J. Strachey, Ed. and Trans.). London: Hogarth Press (Referred to in subsequent references as *Standard Edition*).

Freud, S. (1905[1953]). *Three essays on sexuality*. Standard ed., Vol. 7, pp. 125–243. London: Hogarth Press.

Freud, S. (1914[1957]). *On narcissism: An introduction*. Standard ed., Vol. 14, pp. 67–102. London: Hogarth Press.

Malcolm, J. (1981). *Psychoanalysis: The impossible profession*. New York: Alfred A. Knopf.

Nussbaum, M. (1986). *The fragility of goodness: Luck and ethics in Greek tragedy and philosophy*. Cambridge: Cambridge University Press.

Santas, G. (1988). *Plato and Freud: Two theories of love*. London and New York: Basil Blackwell.

Thompson, M. Guy (2016). On sympathy: The role of love in the therapeutic encounter. *Public Lecture presentation*, Windhorse Foundation, Boulder, CO, September 29.

Chapter 9

Laing and Altered States

Douglas Kirsner, PhD

This chapter introduces and explores Laing's expressed views about altered realities, especially about psychedelics, in particular LSD, using published material as well as the unpublished lectures Laing delivered to the William Alanson White Institute in New York and the New York Academy of Medicine in early 1967.

In 1978 Mick Brown interviewed R. D. Laing for the BBC *Radio Times* in a piece written in relation to the Everyman series *Where Have All the Flowers Gone?* which inquired into whatever happened to the hippies of 1967 (Brown, 1967). Given that Laing was still described as a 'cult hero and observer of the hippies', it is illuminating to see the contrast in how he looked back from the vantage point of 1978 on LSD and the 1960s. Titled 'Acid Test', Mick Brown's article reads in part:

> For most of the period from 1965 to 1970 he was occupied in establishing the Kingsley Hall community in London's East End, where people [Laing said] 'who had got into a state of confused, frantic distress regarded as a type of illness called schizophrenia' could attempt to find a way through their predicament without psychiatric intervention-an experiment that was to have profound effects on psychiatry throughout Europe and America.
>
> It is such work, in psychiatry and related fields of communication, structural anthropology and bio anthropology-little of which came under the scrutiny of the world's media-for which, Laing believes, the 60s will ultimately be remembered. What he calls 'the mediumised view' of the 60s-the spiritual quests and cults, commune living, the search for self realization through meditation-is, he believes, little more than 'transient ephemera' which captured the mind and imagination of the moment.
>
> 'Nothing out of all that was new, except the numbers involved', he says. 'In the history of religious cults and enthusiasms there always seem to crop up these Adventists and Adamites, this thing of loving each other as brothers and sisters in the spirit, and with the plea to give up all personal property and positions, to abolish money and so forth. The 60s had their version of that, in the same way as the 70s have had their version of the Third Awakening in America'. As for LSD, Laing does not believe that its external manifestations have produced anything of lasting cultural significance.

DOI: 10.4324/9781003564294-12

'There is no piece of music, painting, poetry or sculpture that owes its existence to that experience that occurs to me as being memorable'.

As was his wont, Laing was prone to hyperbole. Had he forgotten The Beatles' albums *Revolver* and *Sgt. Pepper?* Or The Doors, Jefferson Airplane and Pink Floyd?

Paul McCartney took John Lennon to the countercultural shop he was involved with, Indica Books and Gallery. There Lennon came across the new book *The Psychedelic Experience: A Manual Based on the Tibetan Book of the Dead* (Leary et al., 2000). Lennon read the entire book in the shop and within days presented the song to The Beatles issued as 'Tomorrow Never Knows', released in 1966. The song begins, 'Turn off your mind, relax and float downstream / It is not dying, it is not dying / Lay down all thoughts, surrender to the void / It is shining, it is shining'.

Brown's article concludes:

The psychedelic revolution was stifled in mid-cry by the simple expedient of making LSD illegal. "If it were still generally available, there would be a lot of people taking it', says Laing. "I don't think that would change the world as the people in Haight-Ashbury believed but it would certainly give a slightly different inflection to things'

(Brown, 1967)

Thus, for Laing, the 1960s would be remembered not for the summers of love, drugs and rock'n'roll but for the advances in psychiatry and communications theory and their applications. During the 1960s prior to his sabbatical in India and Ceylon, Laing was mega-productive, contributing his fundamental and most serious work focusing in detail upon the implications of developments in understanding and articulating the nature of experience and communications between people, examining their contexts, assumptions, ascriptions, distortions, sets, systems and operations.

Laing was intent on questioning the assumptions behind everything, without accepting any 'givens' as unchallengeable. LSD was a means, a tool, in this search and not an end in itself. Its use could provide opportunities in certain settings and conditions for connections with our spiritual side or the cosmos and, crucially, a method of going back behind what he termed 'the cutoff', where we so far repressed aspects of ourselves and our history that these aspects were unavailable and literally unrecognizable.

Laing had a radical concept of who we are. He thought that Freud's division of id, ego and superego, or what can be translated from the German as it, I and over-me, did not really go far enough. Both Freud and Laing were influenced by Groddeck's (1923) book, *The Book of the It* (Groddeck, 1928). In *The Ego and the Id*, Freud (1923) credited Groddeck with the term 'Das Es', the It, for the Id. The motto of *The Ego and the Id* has, unfortunately, been too often translated as 'Where id was ego shall be', which conveys the impression that therapy involves replacing the irrational id with the rational conscious ego. Whereas a truer translation would imply going in the opposite direction: 'Where it was, there I shall be'. That gives the sense of a voyage of discovery into deep inner space. The self-discovery would be of the real 'me' as the apparent 'it' from which our selves emanate. The 'it' is the major ground of our being, and the apparent I or ego forms only a small but of course important proportion of who we are. Laing felt that by calling our inner selves an 'it', this depersonalizes us with a focus on what looks mechanistic instead of being who we are. Like Freud, Laing had a profound conviction of the unconscious running the show, but that unconscious was still both more profound and more personal than Freud proposed.

My chapter on Laing's concept of therapy (Chapter 5) ended with a quotation from Freud that Laing approvingly discussed comparing neurotic struggles with the struggle in neurosis between a polar bear and a whale, which are each on different grounds, footings and levels of terrain. For Freud, neurosis occurs from the clash of a conscious wish battling an unconscious wish, which are on different psychological footings and different levels and resolve each other into symptoms.

Laing took this further. There were not only two levels, but communications theory demonstrated that were series of meta-levels, meta-meta levels and so on not only 'within' one's self but in nonverbal communications between people. Repression, for Laing, involved not just suppression or forgetting but the further operation of forgetting that one has forgotten, so that it is removed from consciousness, like a magic slate. Freud is very much on board thus far with his idea of the 'mystic writing pad' in which censorship occurs on different levels: while one hand is writing letters on it, the other is removing it lifting the waxed page of the pad (Freud, 1925).

For Laing, deeper embedded injunctions and assumptions piled together on top of one another from childhood and in relation to perceptions and injunctions between self and others, particularly in family constellations. Moreover, cultures and societies at large are rife with habitual, taken-for-granted assumptions as givens, all of which result in mystifications and confusions that may need unravelling. However, despite some of Laing's statements that LSD and psychedelics were not intrinsically important, in fact, they clearly helped open his and others' eyes to some significant aspects of present and alternate altered realities.

Laing's own history further explains both the context and philosophy that lay behind his views. He was clearly excited by the potential of LSD to open realms of experience we normally deny ourselves or that are denied to us. He was influenced by writings such as Aldous Huxley's 1954 classic, *The Doors of Perception*, on mescaline and Stanislas Grof's *Realms of the Human Unconscious: Observations from LSD Research*, researched from 1956 onwards in Prague through his visits to Esalen (Grof, 1975). Laing had his first joint, psychedelic mushroom and dose of mescaline and LSD in 1960 at the age of 33, an age, as his son Adrian drily notes, when most people give them up.

By 1966 Laing was fully engaged with taking LSD and other hallucinogens and using them with patients in Kingsley Hall and his practice at 21 Wimpole Street,

London. At Kingsley Hall the philosophy was to find one's true authentic self, and LSD was seen to be part of the way to achieve this goal. The effects of LSD mimicked psychotic breakdown, and breakdown, as Laing famously said, could sometimes be breakthrough. LSD intrigued Laing, and he was given the permission of the Home Office to experiment with it therapeutically. Under the 1964 Misuse of Drugs Act, doctors were entitled to prescribe LSD.

Laing told a very establishment medical conference in 1966, 'the aim of therapy will be to enhance consciousness, not to diminish it. Drugs of choice, if any are to be used, will be predominantly consciousness expanding drugs, rather than consciousness constrictors – the psychic energizers, not the tranquilizers' (cited in A. Laing, 1994, p. 121).

Laing took a small amount of LSD with patients for four- to six-hour sessions, with varying degrees of success. Former patients told Adrian Laing that LSD sessions could be exhilarating and liberating. Some patients found that just one session benefited them more than years of orthodox psychoanalysis, while for others it was too much too soon.

Laing recommended Sean Connery take LSD to deal with the stress of filming *Goldfinger* in the early 1960s. Connery had a bad trip with Laing which was, Connery told Edna O'Brien, a 'freight of terrors' (*The Scotsman*, 2012).

Laing said himself that MDMA (ecstasy) made him feel normal, implying he normally felt somewhat insane . . . or just depressed?

The issue of the controlled use in an appropriate setting versus the uncontrolled use of LSD was crucial. Laing often took a nuanced view of LSD and was generally more responsible about it than he was reputed to be – not a high bar. While Laing generally did not favor the unsupervised use of powerful doses of LSD that could potentially injure patients or others, Adrian Laing observed that Laing's Wimpole Street practice gained mythological status in the 1960s due to the therapeutic use of LSD.

The context is important to understand. Drugs such as opium and heroin were widely used and not previously illegal in many countries around the world. LSD was legal for decades after its sole producer, Sandoz Laboratories, began marketing it in 1947. LSD was introduced into the United States in 1948. During the 1950s it was widely used, and because of its ability to imitate psychosis, its use was even encouraged among undergraduate psychology students and psychiatrists. The period from 1950 and 1965 saw dozens of books, a thousand scientific papers and many international conferences about LSD, and it was prescribed to 40,000 patients. This period was followed by a backlash when it became illegal in certain US states during the mid-1960s. Congressional hearings led to further legislation controlling hallucinogens in the late 1960s. Its illegality increased as it became more popular, especially via the counter-culture. Although the 1960s was the era famous for sex, drugs and rock'n'roll, the 1950s also featured rock'n'roll and quite a few drugs.

Of course, sex took a great leap forward following Food and Drug Administration (FDA) approval for the contraceptive pill in 1960 and blended in rather well with the others. And LSD was produced and distributed in extraordinary and massive quantities during the late 1960s, as you will see in the 2016 movie, *Orange*

Sunshine, and also as pictured in the earlier movie, *The Sunshine Makers*. LSD was banned in California in October 1966 and banned in all states by October 1968 via the Staggers-Dodd Bill.

In the UK, LSD was legal during the 1960s, only becoming restricted to specific prescribers in 1973. In fact, Laing seemed to be unaware of the change in legislation when, in a routine search of his Eton Road house soon after a burglary around 1975, police found some LSD and charged Laing with illegal possession of a Class A drug under the Misuse of Drugs Acts, 1973. Laing managed to get off the charge on the grounds that the prosecution could not prove that the LSD was not purchased prior to 1973 when doctors were permitted to prescribe it.

M. Guy Thompson, who worked with Laing, told me that Laing told the initial meeting of training seminar participants for the Philadelphia Association around 1973 that there should be a minimum of three requirements for therapists in training:

1. To be in full psychoanalysis
2. To read the collected works of Sigmund Freud
3. To sample LSD

Timothy Leary declared, 'LSD is a drug that produces fear in people who don't take it'. In fact, the 2021 Global Drug Survey concluded that psychedelic mushrooms, marijuana and LSD were relatively safe recreational drugs in terms of reporting people seeking emergency medical care over the past year (Global Drug Survey, 2021).

The halcyon days of psychedelic research in the 1950s were followed by a bad trip during the 1960s. But LSD research resumed, and recent research in Europe and the United States has demonstrated that the therapeutic use of psychedelics, including ecstasy, LSD and psilocybin, clearly produce positive outcomes in the treatment of anxiety and depression.

In 1964, Timothy Leary, Richard Alpert (Ram Dass) and Ralph Metzner, wrote:

A psychedelic experience is a journey to new realms of consciousness. The scope and content of the experience is limitless, but its characteristic features are the transcendence of verbal concepts, of space-time dimensions, and of the ego or identity. Such experiences of enlarged consciousness can occur in a variety of ways: sensory deprivation, yoga exercises, disciplined meditation, religious or aesthetic ecstasies, or spontaneously. Most recently they have become available to anyone through the ingestion of psychedelic drugs such as LSD, psilocybin, mescaline, DMT, etc. Of course, the drug does not produce the transcendent experience. It merely acts as a chemical key – it opens the mind, frees the nervous system of its ordinary patterns and structures.

(Leary et al., 2000)

Included in this must-read, fascinating book, *Birth of a Psychedelic Culture*, by Ralph Metzner and Ram Dass is an account by Ram Dass of his encounter with Laing in London where they took LSD together (Mullan, 1995, pp. 221–222).

An amazing part of the context of the mass manufacture and distribution of LSD, or orange sunshine, in the late 1960s was the Brotherhood of Eternal Love. It was set up in Laguna Beach and other parts of California complete with its own spiritual high priest, Tim Leary. The Brotherhood believed they had a spiritual mission to turn on the world. To this end, they manufactured many millions of doses of LSD and smuggled and traded tens of thousands of kilos of hashish and marijuana. Not only the United States and Canada but the UK and Europe were in their empire. Their credibility among buyers was the highest. They saw the world as an insane asylum that they, the lunatics, needed to liberate. Just as Aldous Huxley observed about mescaline, they thought nobody would be the same after they took LSD. Thus, generations of youth could change the world if, as Leary famously put it, they would only 'tune in, turn on and drop out'.

Laing claimed he was offered charge of the operation for the UK and Europe but he refused. He didn't like the generic approach of turning everybody on, regardless of set or setting. LSD could be calibrated as a potent means in conjunction with a suitable guide and adapted to the individual situation and needs but was scarcely a panacea in itself for Laing. To the contrary, it could be dangerous. The plan to turn on Berkeley Haight Ashbury youth with 300,000 units of LSD appalled Laing. In any event, low-cost mass doses of LSD were distributed and bought by the generation around the United States, the UK and Europe, obviously particularly in California (Mullan, 1995, pp. 222–226).

In case anyone might think that Laing might have made this up, that Timothy Leary was not in on this approach or that it was only the Brotherhood of Eternal Love that acted to spread the joy, I quote from the book, *Orange Sunshine: The Brotherhood of Eternal Love and the Quest to Spread Peace, Love and Acid in the World* by Nicholas Schou:

> On February 14, 1968, Timothy Leary granted an interview to a reporter with the *Long Beach Press Telegram*. It was Valentine's Day and Leary wanted the world to know that he was now dedicating his life to bringing love to the masses – one acid trip at a time. 'A great breakthrough in evolution is under way, a drastic change in the way men think', the paper quoted Leary in a story that ran the next morning. 'We have dedicated men who manufacture LSD and other psychedelics and release them under controlled circumstances in given arenas to see what will happen. One million doses were released recently in the Haight Ashbury district in San Francisco – the most ever released in one place at one time so far, but there are men who can release up to 10 million doses at a time. Leary refused to answer the reporter's questions about who was making all that LSD and insisted that he and his unnamed accomplices were motivated purely by a desire to change the world. 'We're not out to amass great sums of money – we need only enough to support the work we're doing', he said. 'When we need it, it is there. The Lord provides'.

(Schou, 2011, p. 147)

This is how Laing himself responded to these events. Laing recalls:

I was absolutely appalled by it . . . Leary and Alpert had thought about this plan to distribute something like 300,000 acid trips within a 24 hour period too late school college and first year university students.

Sometime after that Alpert came over to have a chat and get my reactions to things and he put to me. . . . He said that they regarded Europe as my territory, and Britain in particular. They would like to do this to London, what they have done in Berkeley. But, he said, we regard London and England, Scotland and Europe – but they have no real concept of Europe, they were thinking of Chelsea – as your territory and if you say no, that's the end of it . . . so I said, well, if you are asking me, well, no. they said fine, okay, and that was an end to it. So they never carried out that operation they had done in Berkeley and San Francisco on the school children and 17-year-olds of London. They said fine, okay, and that was an end to it.

I thought it was an incredible arrogance to think of themselves as some sort of world command. I mean on unsuspecting people without telling them what they were letting themselves in for, and to missionize this. I thought it was just another symptom of the disease that they were purporting to address and to cure.

If one had time to go easy on this and really working out, it could be a really useful therapeutic agent. But it needed quietness and a lack of hysteria over a period of time to begin to get the hang of how this could be employed.

(Mullan, 1995, p. 222)

However, I suspect that the Brotherhood of Eternal Love simply gave up on him, bypassed him and moved on to other distributors. The extent of their deep reach across and within nations could not be clearer when you view the extraordinary film *Orange Sunshine* (2016), based on interviews with members of the Brotherhood. At the very least, they had a quasi-religious mission to fulfil. Laing contacted the British Home Office and spoke with Scotland Yard about it, all to no avail (Mullan, 1995, p. 225).

Laing was on a serious quest to understand the human world. Clearly, he also loved to have fun. For decades he was no stranger to alcohol, nor from the age of 33 in 1960 to drugs. Psychedelic drugs, particularly mescaline and LSD, were for him means of both enjoyment and enlightenment of himself and others. But his use of them with others, whether at Kingsley Hall or his practice in Wimpole Street, was primarily as a therapeutic aid together with being a research aid for opening up experience.

At that time, the experience of a metanoiac voyage was seen as desirable, even essential, both as part of the Kingsley Hall experiment and more widely. The term 'metanoia' is Greek for 'repentance' but literally 'change of mind'. The term 'paranoia' means 'beside mind (*noos*)'. Metanoia involves a transformative change of mind, as in repentance. Like love, as Andrew Lloyd Webber might have said, it changes everything, including behavior, change of heart, even conversion.

In a lecture titled 'Metanoia' in 1968, Laing proposed two hypotheses:

1. Schizophreniform breakdown may be a resource called upon when all else seems impossible.
2. If the set and setting can be changed, the experience may be so transformed that it may no longer need to be regarded as 'psychotic' at all (R. D. Laing, 1972, pp. 11–12).

LSD was originally regarded as a psychotomimetic substance, that is, producing in the mind effects similar to psychosis. Laing saw it as having a natural analogue in a metanoiac voyage. The nature of this voyage was dependent on the set and setting. Mental hospitals define that voyage as madness per se and treat it accordingly. According to Laing, the setting of a psychiatric clinic promotes in staff and patients the set best designed to turn the metanoiac voyage from a voyage of discovery into self of a potentially revolutionary and liberating nature into what he called a 'catastrophe: into a pathological process from which the person requires to be cured' (R. D. Laing, 1972, p. 12).

Laing told his audience in his William Alanson White lectures that in the New Testament,

> Repentance or metanoia, change of mind, was related to what was called baptism. John the Baptist baptizing people in the water and saying that someone would come, greater than him, who were baptized people not only in water but in fire and in air. Baptism means apparently something like an inversion, a cleansing a sort of death prior to a rebirth. Both repentance and baptism closely interwoven into that sequence of returning to the womb and being born again, and thereby changing from the old man to the new man.
>
> Metanoia as a term that would simply mean a change of mind of this particular time, of going into meta-experiential realms, all domains of experience beyond our cut-off from them, going to a variable distance in those meta regions of experience, and eventually returning; the experience of the return as a natural experience, frequently, of a sort of rebirth.
>
> A metanoiac voyage, or process, would entail some measure of initiation into those regions of our potential experience, or of our mind, or what is of being, which is beyond our normal range, without any presupposition on our part in using such a term that there's anything at all pathological about this, but rather that the state of engulfment in the body of our own death whereby we're asleep and don't know that we're asleep, so forgetful that we can't even remember that we've forgotten, so ignorant that we don't even know that we don't know, that is the condition that this process, fundamentally speaking, has the function of awakening us from.

> (R. D. Laing, 1967c)

In his address to the first International Rochester Conference on the Origins of Schizophrenia in March 1967, Laing says,

> The metanoiac sequence lends itself to the metaphor of a voyage inwards and backwards, until it reaches a turning point, and the voyager returns through an accelerated neogenesis, forwards, once more, and outwards into the world without loss of self . . . it appears to be a sort of death rebirth sequence, from which if successfully negotiated, the person returns to the world feeling new born, refreshed, and re-integrated at a higher level of functioning than before.
>
> (R. D. Laing, 1967a, pp. 141–142)

Laing thought there was a taboo on moving backward, but it was often a precondition for moving forwards. Thus, a voyage was then going backwards to go forwards, and regression was a condition of progression. Regression was a term Freud used for a return to a more primitive point, a reversion to past phases of development both temporally and structurally.

This leads to the heart of what lay behind Laing's interest in LSD for the therapeutic process. For Laing, the place of LSD in therapy was that of a chemical enabler. It provided the opportunity to produce regression and reversion to earlier experiences that were unconscious, many of which were made unconscious through various operations both that others had induced and we induced upon ourselves. This was especially so for the experiences that we forget, but those that we forget that we have forgotten, the levels of the system that gave us the illusion that what we now remember or experience is all that exists, and that there are no realms that we have forgotten because we have forgotten that we have forgotten.

In Chapter 5 I discussed Laing's view of therapy as centering upon mystification. Mystification involved something akin to a hypnotic suggestion or a spell cast that needed to be revealed and then, if possible, countermanded and counter-suggested.

In line with Laing's theory about hypnotic suggestion and the spells or unconscious injunctions that are wrought on us or by us, could it be that LSD or the psychedelics could take us back behind the original suggestion so that the slate is wiped clean and a new suggestion, counter-suggestion or no suggestion can be made to the extent that we are hard programmed? Perhaps psychedelics could help a reset. Or to extend the analogy, even perform a reboot or reconfiguration to factory settings. Laing discussed some of these issues about operations and our being hard programmed in his White lectures.

Therapy could involve going back through levels of reality that constructed a person's present psychic world, making the current consensual version of reality seem a self-evident, unchallengeable given. After we have forgotten that we have forgotten, LSD could pierce through and behind these barriers of illusory givens to see them in context as constructions. Once they are seen as constructions, there are therefore alternative scenarios that a person can choose, or at least understand why they haven't taken them. As Laing told Bob Mullan:

> There was a lot to think about in the relationship of the altered states of mind that acid put you into and the way people got confused and lost and shipwrecked in psychotic states of misery. How could they get out of it? Was there a possibility that acid could release someone from being caught in the hell [world] and allow a movement to occur, which they might, in the presence of other people, move themselves back into a balanced, sane world, if they've ever been in it before?
>
> (Mullan, 1995, p. 226)

Laing asserts that the theory of regression is going back in time, beyond the false self and what one has done to oneself and where one lost oneself, to begin again. 'In order to get back to a state of unintegration, a person has to frequently regress in time. The most frequently missed function of regression . . . is to undergo, a method of undoing repression' (R. D. Laing, 1967c).

From the beginning in *The Divided Self* in 1960, Laing assumes we are always agents, or persons who have intentions. We are not things or mechanisms. Therefore, understanding our actions and behavior becomes a function of never giving up that premise to, for example, mechanistic explanations or victim explanations which exclude personal intention. This includes obviously behaviorism but also the kind of general biological, sociological or cultural reductionist explanations. For Laing, human intention and meaning are always part of the behavior of a person or persons.

Thus, we can explain human behavior in personal, existential terms. That is fine for conscious behavior. It is also understandable for pre-conscious and even the levels of unconscious behavior that Freud revealed, initially in his dream theory, and then in his psychopathology of everyday life, theories of anxiety and neurosis. We don't know how much we don't know. Freud began to understand the operations of human intentions on ourselves and others – he was a hero of the voyages into the underworld, as Laing wrote early. Freud also began to explain the operations we carry out on ourselves and others, those we attribute to one another, often unknowingly, especially to ourselves.

Laing is convinced that an inner journey which takes our individual experience seriously would provide access to a stranger world than exploration of the external world could achieve. Laing suggests that we need to take a different direction and take it to be valid experience. As he puts it,

> One person investigating the experience of another can be fully aware only of his own experience of the other. He cannot have direct awareness of the other's experience of the 'same' world. He cannot see through the other's eyes and cannot hear through the other's ears. The only true voyage, Proust once remarked, would be not to travel through a hundred different lands with the same pair of eyes but to see the same land through a hundred different pairs of eyes. All one

'feels', 'senses', 'intuits'; etc. of the other entails inference from one's own experience of the other to the other's experience of one's self.

(R. D. Laing, 1981, p. 28. See Proust, 2000, p. 291)

This theme of the inner voyage is very much at the forefront of Laing's most famous and best-known book, *The Politics of Experience and the Bird of Paradise* (1967b), which saw those labeled mad to be sufficiently 'out of formation' to enable them to be explorers of the inner world. I believe Laing's overall or 'global project', as Sartre might have called it, was to begin to provide a thoroughgoing personal account of experience and behavior in human terms. So that involved challenging 'givens' at every stage. 'Mad' behavior and actions might make some sense, especially from the 'mad' person's point of view. Laing strongly rejected Karl Jaspers' conviction that psychosis was a barrier and is 'un-understandable' (Jaspers, 1997, p. 577), believing that psychosis was far more understandable than was often assumed and might sometimes provide a further pathway, perhaps a break in the wall, to understanding human beings in general.

Trying to understand psychosis, Laing increasingly tried to lay bare the operators or operations on experience, both by self and by others, and to understand the interweaving of these operations inside, between or beside ourselves. So that meant bracketing out or challenging taken-for-granted basic assumptions – givens. These operations on experience include repression, identification, projection, introjection, denial, regression and splitting.

On a direct horizontal level, Laing examined self-other and family or group interactions that define our realities, using theories such as Gregory Bateson's double-bind theory and Sartre's theories about series and nexus.

But there are also the vertical and deeper, historical, experiential operations beneath and levels of awareness at many levels that deny each other and interweave. So Laing questions reality at every level and sees LSD as a means of fast-tracking regression and insight, as it were, cutting out the resistant middleman!

Laing owed a tremendous debt to Freud and took the spirit of his writings very seriously. Freud revealed some levels of cutoffs and also the operations of experience. For Freud, the unconscious world whose content is representative of the drives is governed by primary processes, especially by condensation and displacement. Our consciousness was a small part of who we are for Freud, who took on Groddeck's theory of *Das Es*, the It. Laing believed that the It went still deeper, seeming to be alien and controlling us, but in fact a central part of us that we need to make our own in a consistently personal psychology. As Laing puts it in the White lectures,

It's only from a remarkably socially relative position of alienation that our essential true selves we take to be the id. The id is us – it's the id that's doing it all despite us is not the it – it's precisely who we are. It's because we pitched out to ourselves that we talk about the small fragment of our total being as our ego, and our fundamental being as though it were something else. Many people even doubt that we have our selves. By the time we've lost ourselves so completely as that, we're so depersonalized that we don't even know that we're depersonalized.

(R. D. Laing, 1967c)

Laing explains:

It's not our unconscious that's unconscious, but our consciousness that we identify ourselves with, which is only a small fragment of our mind, is unconscious of our consciousness. It's not the unconscious that's unconscious; it's we that are unconscious of our unconsciousness.

(R. D. Laing, 1967c)

The cutoffs or barriers that we don't see in ourselves are important if only because they don't appear to exist. But this is illusory, even if many people in our current society don't question it. Laing was fond of saying that when viewed through history and cultural anthropology, very few outside the current generation would think of our current scene as normal. In his lecture at the New York Academy of Medicine, January 9, 1967, Laing proposes that when we look horizontally across all cultures and vertically back four or five generations,

There might be no one . . . who sees what's going on. If anyone comes through with a statement about what is going on, they are in very considerable jeopardy. There's very little relationship in this whole world between what is going on and what people say is going on.

(Laing, 1967c)

Reality, normal or altered, as Laing would so often say, is always 'up for grabs'.

References

Brown, M. (1967). Acid test. *Radio Times*, January 19.

Dass, R. and Metzner, R. (2010). *Birth of a psychedelic culture*. Santa Fe: Synergetic.

Freud, S. (1923). The ego and the id. In J. Strachey (ed.), *The standard edition of the complete psychological works of Sigmund Freud*, Vol. XIX (1923–1925): The ego and the id and other works, pp. 1–66. London: Hogarth Press.

Freud, S. (1925). A note upon 'the mystic writing-pad'. In J. Strachey (ed.), *The standard edition*, Vol. XIX (1923–1925): The ego and the id and other works, pp. 227–232. London: Hogarth Press.

Global Drug Survey (2021). www.globaldrugsurvey.com/wp-content/uploads/2021/12/Report2021_global.pdf

Groddeck, G. (1928). *The book of the it: Psychoanalytic letters to a friend*. New York: Nervous and Mental Disease Publishing Co.

Grof, S. (1975). *Realms of the human unconscious: Observations from LSD research*. New York: Viking Press.

Jaspers, K. (1997). *General psychopathology* (J. Hoenig and M. W. Hamilton, Trans.). Baltimore, MD: Johns Hopkins University Press.

Laing, A. (1994). *R. D. Laing: A biography*. London: Peter Owen.

Laing, R. D. (1967a). Family and social contexts in relation to the origin of schizophrenia. In J. Romano (ed.), *Proceedings of the first Rochester International Conference on Schizophrenia*, March 29–31, Excerpta Medica, International Conference Series, no. 151, Amsterdam, pp. 139–145.

Laing, R. D. (1967b). *The politics of experience and the bird of paradise*. Harmondsworth: Penguin Books.

Laing, R. D. (1967c). *Lectures to William Alanson White Institute and the New York Academy of Medicine*. Unpublished transcript.

Laing, R. D. (1972). Metanoia: Some experiences at Kingsley Hall, London. In H. Ruitenbeek (ed.), *Going crazy: The radical therapy of R D Laing and others*, pp. 11–25. New York: Bantam Books.

Laing, R. D. (1981). *Self and others*. Harmondsworth: Penguin Books.

Leary, T., Metzner, R., and Alpert, R. (2000). *The psychedelic experience: A manual based on The Tibetan book of the dead*. London: Penguin Books.

Mullan, R. (1995). *Mad to be normal: Conversations with RD Laing*. London: Free Association Books.

Proust, M. (2000). *In search of lost time, volume V: The captive, the fugitive*. New York: Vintage.

Schou, N. (2011). *Orange sunshine: The brotherhood of eternal love and the quest to spread peace love and acid in the world*. New York: Thomas Dunne Books St Martin's Press.

The Scotsman (2012). September 24. www.scotsman.com/news/celebrity/sir-sean-connery-took-lsd-with-rd-laing-irish-author-1-2543769

IV

What Is Love?

Chapter 10

Eros and Agapè

M. Guy Thompson, PhD

Introduction

The word "love" means so many things in different contexts that to try a general and all-encompassing definition is probably impossible. The topic of love is also one of the most pervasive in Laing's published works, as well as his lectures and private seminars. It was Laing's many allusions to Christianity over the years and the way some of its principal tenets influenced his thinking that inspired this essay.

For the purposes of this chapter, I want to address one of Laing's most frequent allusions to love, *caritas*, in the context of Christianity. Though I won't be citing Laing explicitly, I will be alluding to a favorite expression of Laing's that he invoked often – "the heart of the matter" – that epitomizes the underlying theme of this chapter. In fact, the *heart* of the matter, when we speak of the human condition, would necessarily allude to the role love plays in our lives – for what is closer to our hearts than love?

My aim is to explore the relation between two Greek words for love, **eros** and **agapé**, by comparing and contrasting the two in relation to a Latin term for love coined by Augustine, **caritas**, which, as we will see, integrates *eros* and *agapé*. However, there are at least eight words for love in the Greek language, and probably more. **Eros** is the most familiar, referring to erotic or passionate love. *Philia* refers to friendship, or affection. *Storge* refers to family or familiar love. *Ludus* depicts playful or teasing love. *Mania*[1] is obsessive or mad love. *Pragma* is enduring or marital love. *Philautia* is narcissistic or self-love, but in the positive sense of the term. And finally *agapé* is selfless or spiritual love. I want to focus specifically on the first and last of these variations of love.

But before turning our attention to the relation between *eros* and *agapé*, I want to say something about two other closely related kinds of love: *philia* and *storge*. These are sometimes conflated. For example, some people refer to *philia* as brotherly or sisterly love, as Laing himself sometimes did, perhaps because in Christianity, friendship and brotherhood are closely related, if only metaphorically. This is not technically accurate. Strictly speaking, *philia* refers to non-erotic as well as non-kinship love. Unlike familial love, we choose whom we decide to become friends with. We are born into our familial relationships, represented in the Greek

DOI: 10.4324/9781003564294-14

idiom as *storge*. This is why love among siblings, parents and children, uncles and aunts and so on are *familiar* to us. We don't choose these relationships; we're born into them by blood or marriage.

Aristotle believed that friendship is the most intimate love. We are drawn to friends by an attraction that Freud believed is partially erotic but not sexualized as in the case of genital intercourse. Freud's view that friendships are erotic but not sexual is indebted entirely to Plato. The fact that friendships are not rooted in sex is what makes them so special. They thrive on reciprocity and embody a capacity for give-and-take that is often missing in sexual relationships, which are governed by passion. As we will see, Christianity reveres friendship and views it as an edition of *agapé*, the love of and for God.

Storge is not exclusively limited to family relations, but refers to virtually any relationship that is familiar (Lewis, 2012, pp. 31–56). In the same way that we develop feelings for family members over time, we also develop feelings for any people or place that becomes an aspect of our daily routine. A city, for example, that I grew up in has a special hold on me, even though I like to complain about the traffic, the cost of living, or the smog. The stores I shop in, the people who service my needs, the bridge I drive over to work are all familiar to me and become increasingly so over time. Eventually, if I live somewhere long enough, my affection for the place sneaks up on me and I can't help but form an attachment, even if I don't especially like the place. In a word, it becomes home to me, and wherever I live, I long to feel at home. Familiarity is what makes this edition of love sublime. Just like a marriage or a friendship that has lost its magic, I remain attached to it, nonetheless. Anyone who has lived in a variety of places knows what I'm talking about.

Now for the relationship between *eros* and *agapé*. This essay is divided into three sections. The first concerns the mythology of *eros* and *agapé*. The second addresses Plato's conception of *eros*. And finally, in the third section I explore the Christian appropriation of *agapé* and the relationship between *eros*, *agapé*, and *caritas*.

The Myth of *Eros* and *Agapé*

Where does *Eros* belong in Greek mythology? And *Agapé*? First we have to account for *Aphrodite*, the goddess of love. In fact, there are two Greek goddesses of love: *Aphrodite* and *Agapé*. Aphrodite is the goddess of sexual love and Agapé is the goddess of divine love, which we know very little about. But first Aphrodite. She is the goddess of sex, beauty, pleasure, and procreation. In Greek mythology, Aphrodite was married to Hephaestus, the god of blacksmiths and metalworking. Yet Aphrodite had many lovers. Among them was Ares, the god of war. Other lovers included the shepherd Adonis, another shepherd Anchises, and many, many others. It was Aphrodite's feud with two other goddesses that started the Trojan War. Aphrodite was stunningly beautiful, but the Spartans also depicted her as bearing arms, so she was prayed to when they went into battle. Perhaps this is where the phrase, "all is fair in love and war," originated? Aphrodite was also the patron goddess to prostitutes, and many Greek courtesans wrote poems to her.

Now Aphrodite had a special relationship with Eros, who in mythology was sometimes depicted as the god of lust and sexual desire. From a cosmological perspective, Hesiod describes Eros as one of the four primeval forces at the beginning of time. First there was Chaos, or the Void, the first thing to exist. Then came Gaia, the Earth. After Gaia came Tartarus, where souls are judged after death, also known as the Abyss, that became the dungeon where the Titans were imprisoned. And finally there was Eros, love, the fairest of the gods who ruled over the minds of both gods and mortals. Eros was one of the fundamental causes in the formation of the world and brought order and harmony to the conflicting elements of which Chaos consisted. In Plato's *Symposium* he is referred to as the oldest of the gods.

Later, the Greek poets humanized Eros by suggesting he was one of the youngest gods. In this context he was sometimes described as the son of Poros and Penia, resource and need, respectively, and was begotten on Aphrodite's birthday. Others suggest he is the son of Hermes and Aphrodite, while others still insist he is the son of Ares and Aphrodite. This is what is maddening about Greek mythology: there are so many versions of virtually every mythological figure, none of which are definitive. But since love finds its way into the hearts of humans in a manner that no one can fathom, it stands to reason his origin is mysterious.

In art, Eros is always depicted as a handsome youth. He is the god of sensual love and passion, which is much broader than sex. His arms consist of arrows, which he carries in a golden quiver. Some are golden and kindle love in the hearts they wound, while others are made of lead and destroy a love that already existed. He is sometimes represented with golden wings, fluttering like a bird. At other times he is depicted with his eyes covered, and he acts blindly. He is usually the companion to Aphrodite, unreservedly devoted to her, always at the ready to carry out her instructions, for good or ill.

Finally, a few words about the goddess Agapé. She is virtually ignored by Plato and Aristotle, as well as every other Greek philosopher, so all we know about her in the specifically Greek context is her mythology. As I noted a moment ago, she is the goddess of divine love. She is also Aphrodite's sister. Agapé was idolized by all the women in ancient Greece because she refused to give in to any man's orders. Perhaps she was the first feminist? Greek women never saw themselves as very important, even in marriages. This wasn't so for Agapé. She knew that men felt superior to women, but she saw no evidence of their alleged supremacy. She vowed to be an independent goddess and to never let any man or god lie to her. As years went by Agapé became lonely but discovered that she had stopped aging and became increasingly sensuous and beautiful. The gods took notice and tried to seduce her, but they only made fools of themselves in the process. Mortal women began to realize that men weren't the only power in the universe and that women could make decisions of their own. Greek women began to achieve a higher marital status and were treated more fairly. This only made Greek men more attracted to them and less likely to break their marital vows. One wonders why Greek philosophers – all men – have so little to say about her.

Eros and the Divine: Plato

I could say more about the other Greek gods that are associated with love, but given the space, I will move on. I now turn to Plato and what he taught us about love, a composite of Eros's philosophical, psychological, and spiritual aspects.

Plato is generally regarded as the most important of the Greek philosophers. That status could arguably go to Socrates, Plato's teacher and central character in Plato's many dialogues. But Socrates wrote nothing, and most of what we know about him comes from Plato. Consequently, separating which portion of Plato's dialogues belong to Socrates and in turn Plato himself is virtually impossible. This is why you sometimes hear Socrates invoked and other times Plato when describing our debt to the Greeks. Plato not only invented philosophy as we know it; he was also an essential inspiration for Christianity, located in the Christian conceptions of love and the hereafter. Plato was also Aristotle's teacher, the other Greek philosopher who altered the course of history and who founded science. Whereas Plato focused on *eros*, Aristotle turned his attention to *philia* and taught us nearly all that we know about friendship. Plato and Aristotle each had a fundamental impact on Freud and are the source for most of Freud's theories about the human condition.

So what, according to Plato, was *eros*? *Eros* is not only passionate or romantic love but also desire in all its aspects. To desire anything is strictly speaking "erotic." Plato explores *eros* in two of his most famous dialogues, *The Symposium* and *Phaedrus*. *The Symposium* (1991) details a gathering of Socrates and some of his friends and students who met to debate the nature of love – in much the way I am doing in this essay – in both its beautiful and darker aspects. According to Sophocles, "Love is unconquered in battle, sleeps on the maiden's cheek and roams in savage places, whom neither men nor immortals can flee; and who introduces madness and forcibly turns the minds of just men to injustice and their disgrace"(Allen, in Plato, 1991, p. 7).

In the *Hippolytus*, Euripides tells us how "Eros bewitches the heart of those he would destroy. He is the author of ruin, tyrannical in violence, destruction on his breath" (Allen, p. 7–8). And even Plato, who organized this gathering to sing *eros*'s praises, has to admit that "*Eros* is also the master passion of the tyrant . . . and of unsatisfied longing, allied to drunkenness and a source of insanity" (p. 8). So *eros* is not all lovey-dovey. There is a dark side to *eros* as well, which explains why love can be so painful and make us so crazy we may be driven to murder or suicide.

According to Plato, Aphrodite represents sex, whereas Eros represents love, broadly speaking. According to Aristophanes, one of the guests at the *Symposium*, *eros* is the desire for wholeness, embodied in sexual intercourse. This explains why we crave proximity to those we love: we want to be with them and enjoy their company, always and in all ways. Love is possessive and, in that respect, egocentric, a pervasive theme in Freud's theory of narcissism, in both its good and pathogenic aspects.[2]

Keep in mind that the fundamental purpose of philosophy, according to Plato, is to acquire happiness, or *eudaimonia* – literally to be with your *daimon* spirit. In other words, to be with your *daimon* and not banished from his favor will bring happiness. In this context, love is essential to happiness, not just sexual love, but the love of friends, of work, of the seasons, of life itself. This brings us to Eros's origin and whether he was in fact a god or a *daimon* spirit, an entity somewhere between god and man.

The key figure in *The Symposium* is a woman, Diotima, who doesn't actually attend the meeting, but whose wisdom about the nature of love is invoked by Socrates, who professes to know little about love himself. So it is a woman who Socrates – or Plato – turns to as the ultimate authority on the nature of love. According to Diotima, Eros is a *daimon*, an intermediate between gods and mortals. When Aphrodite wants to reward a mortal with love, she dispatches Eros to make it so. Eros is also a philosopher, the first lover of wisdom.

Diotima tells us that Eros is the child of Penia, meaning want or need, and Poros, meaning resourcefulness. This explains love's neediness, its aim to possess, its love of wisdom, and its cunning. Despite the adage that only fools fall in love, Diotima argues that only the wise are able to love fully and unreservedly, to give themselves to love's call completely. She suggests that if love makes us happy, only the wise are capable of genuine happiness when compared to its inferior cousin, pleasure.

But what is happiness? Diotima explains that happiness consists of the possession of good things. The lover loves beauty, for example. For Plato, the good and beauty are the same principle. Happiness is not an episodic experience of pleasure – the way we typically invoke this term – but a state of well-being that persists. The happy individual may also experience suffering from time to time, but as a fundamentally happy person. Happiness doesn't inoculate us from suffering, but it does make it bearable. In the English language, the root of the word happiness is *hap*, meaning luck or chance. But good fortune isn't blind. For Plato, it only comes to those who earn it, by aspiring to become wise and valuing the good. It was Plato who gave us ethics and who combined the ethical with our capacity to love. Basically, the good person is a loving person. The bad person is hateful.

In fact, Plato insists that all desires are ostensibly good and that we only desire bad things out of ignorance, when we mistakenly believe that wishing someone ill, for example, will make us happy. But ultimately it won't, because to wish such a thing would be envy, not love. The satisfaction we derive from vengeance is only momentary and corrupts the soul. This means that *eros* is both sensual and divine. It begins in sexual attraction but aims at something higher. The love of beauty, sexual desire, the aesthetic perfection of the athlete, art objects, or ideas, experienced sensually and examined rationally, leads us to the divine. This is the essence of erotic love, and, borrowing heavily from Plato, it is also how Freud conceived psychoanalysis: a process in which we submit to the dark side of our soul by recounting our sins and then examining them without judgment for the truths they tell us about ourselves. Armed with this knowledge, we have the opportunity to make ourselves better by becoming less defensive and loving more fully.

In distinguishing between love and desire, Plato explained that love is simply a desire that we want to treasure forever. To lose someone's love is the most grievous pain possible, but to lose one's passion for living is even worse. This is why it is in our nature to love, and if we can parse out the obstacles that stand in our way, our capacity for love will only increase. Plato also believed in the hereafter, a notion adopted by Christianity, and argued that if we die as loving creatures, we will go to heaven and live there forever. This is why love, or *eros*, is also divine. After all, it leads us to heaven. But for the Greeks, we must find this heaven on earth, before we die, or we will go to Hades.

We can see from this brief description that Plato conceived *eros* as all-encompassing. Yet Aristotle, in his *Nicomachean Ethics* (2000), thought there was something missing. He turned his attention to *philia*, which he thought was an even more loving, more giving edition of *eros*. This love is not different in kind from *eros*, but rather an extension of it. Because it is inherently reciprocal, it is due to our capacity for *philia* that we are willing to forgive others for their trespasses against us. Any person we love is also capable of wounding us, and often does. The good friend overlooks these intransigencies and remains loyal. A friend doesn't judge harshly, but feels sympathy for the shortcomings of those he or she befriends. This is the element in marriages that ensures their longevity. We will see how this conception of friendship had just as great an impact on Christianity as did *eros*.

Agapé and Caritas

During the early period of Christianity, from the death of Christ to the formation of the Roman Catholic Church in the fourth century, Christianity was composed of competing churches that were influenced by both Plato's conception of *eros* and the teachings of Christ, as articulated by the four Gospels of John, Mark, Luke, and Matthew, but especially St. Paul's Corinthians. Christ himself was schooled in Greek thought, as all educated Jews were. Yet St. Paul, who lived in the first century after the death of Jesus, was singularly opposed to sex as well as any aspect of *eros* that was even tangentially erotic. This is why many of the early gospels were excluded from official Christendom when the New Testament was collated, especially the Gospel of Thomas that was thought to be too Platonic.

It was Paul who introduced the language of *agapé* into Christ's teachings as epitomizing Christian love, though the word employed in the King James translation from the Greek is either love or charity (a corruption of *caritas*). In the original Greek, the term *agapé* is employed.

So how does Paul conceptualize *agapé*, and how does he distinguish it from *eros*? In Paul's opinion, *agapé* is the opposite of *eros*. Whereas *eros* is epitomized by man's love for God and situated in a split between the carnal and the divine (which can be elevated through good deeds and self-development), *agapé* is epitomized by God's love for man, *in spite of his sinful ways*, which God accepts as his nature. Because many early Christians remained influenced by Platonic love, Paul set out to oppose it in a variety of edicts.

Whereas Plato taught that the universe is of one substance, Christianity teaches a radical disjunction between man and God. Whereas Plato emphasized that man can employ reason to examine and improve himself, Jesus preaches that salvation comes from faith. Whereas *eros* values sexual energy in its various forms and teaches that desire for a lover can train the soul to love more magnanimously, Christianity treats sex with suspicion and advocates the control of our sexual urges. For Plato, evil derives from ignorance and can be corrected; for Christianity, humans are fallen creatures who rely on God's forgiveness for their salvation. For the Greeks, ethics derives from shame and one's place in the community. For Christians, ethics is rooted in the guilt of having been born in sin, from the consequence of Adam and Eve. Only God can forgive us for this original sin.

Plato implies that *eros* contains elements of *agapé* within it, in the guise of *philia*. As we saw earlier, *eros* was never supposed to be exclusively sexual. It wasn't until Christianity that *eros* was separated from *philia* and *agapé*, thereby demeaning *eros* as self-centered and lustful, while elevating p*hilia* and *agapé* to a selfless, sexless conception of love.

How have these changes in this conception of love impacted the history of Christianity? Three centuries after Paul, Augustine, a North African Greek born in Carthage in the fourth century, tried to integrate the competing visions of love that were still being debated: *eros* derived from Plato; *agapé* derived from Paul. Augustine is responsible for bringing Plato's conception of love into Christianity as a legitimate and enduring presence.

Because many fourth-century Christians embraced Paul's conception of *agapé* and resisted efforts to include any mention of Plato's *eros*, Augustine cannily introduced a new term, the Latin *caritas*, to sneak in Plato's concept of love. By replacing *agapé* with *caritas*, Augustine was able to avoid the appearance of relying too explicitly on the Greeks. The central idea, following Plato, is that all humans seek *eudaimonia* as their goal in life and their quest for the "highest good." Rejecting the notion that humans are rooted in sin and rely exclusively on God's grace, Augustine argues that we have a more active role in our salvation. He suggests that all love is acquisitive and that we desire to possess the object of our love in order to ensure happiness. This conception of love is Platonic in its essence. So how does he reconcile this interpretation of *eros* with Paul's notion of *agapé*?

As with Plato, Augustine says it all depends on the *object* of desire as to whether that desire is good or bad. But because we all aim for what is good in life, the ultimate good must be God. Because we are composed of both body and spirit, we are capable of loving worldly objects – *cupiditas* – which is sinful, as well as those that are divinely sanctioned. If our love for God is strong and we are able to receive His love in turn, we will embrace *caritas* instead. This will lead to redemption – Augustine's term for happiness. Even when we desire evil, there is nonetheless a small element in that evil that is good. Following Plato, Augustine suggests we have merely misled ourselves when succumbing to evil desires but have it within us to correct our folly and seek the good instead. True happiness depends on seeking the "right" good. In this formulation, God's grace, so essential to the Christian conception of *agapé*, is retained, though diminished in importance. Whereas Christians emphasize God's love of mankind as the source of their salvation, Augustine, following the Neoplatonists, emphasizes man's love for God, rooted in a passionate and egocentric love for himself as well as for other human beings. And because we are mortal, we are assured that our love of God will persist after we die for all eternity, when we join Him in Heaven.

The distinctive feature of Augustine's conception of *caritas*, which embraces both *eros* and *agapé*, is its giving, generous nature. To love fully is a giving of oneself to the other, suspending all judgment and criticism, while blinding oneself to any sinful qualities that reside in the love object. It is a love that is both forgiving and altruistic, reflecting the love God feels for mortal creatures, not selflessly, but *passionately*. Unlike Paul, Augustine insisted that to love God fully must contain elements of passion. Otherwise, it would be love without a soul.

Nearly a thousand years later, just as Augustine sneaked Plato into Christianity, Thomas Aquinas, the thirteenth-century monk, ushered in Aristotle. It was Aquinas who emphasized the "brotherhood" of Christianity and defined *caritas* explicitly as a friendship between man and God. Now all Christians were "brothers-in-arms" and friendship became something inherently divine. During the thousand years between Augustine and Aquinas, Europe endured a period of history known as the Middle Ages, the era between ancient and modern history. There was perpetual chaos and intrigue as competing monks, priests, popes, and other believers fought over the definition of Christianity. Yet Europe flourished until the Dark Ages, when Islam displaced the Roman Empire and eventually ended Byzantium, when the Muslims took Constantinople. The competition between *eros* and *agapé* persisted throughout this period, but for the most part, the Platonic influence prevailed. This culminated in the Renaissance, a period of unsurpassed prosperity and secular enlightenment that brought Europe into the modern era. Obviously this couldn't last.

A backlash finally occurred when Pietro de Medici fled Italy and the Italian Dominican friar, Girolamo Savonarola, seized power. In four brief years he wreaked havoc over Florentine society and set fire to paintings, books, and other treasures that he insisted were tainted by Greek influence. This was thankfully short-lived, and after Savonarola was himself burned at the stake, the Medicis returned to power and sanity again prevailed. Though the Renaissance survived, the damage that Savonarola generated left its mark. The Catholic Church suffered one disaster after another with a succession of corrupt popes that culminated in reforms both within and outside the Vatican. The Reformation was around the corner, and *agapé* would once again gain ascendency.

Something had to give. Disgusted with both a corrupt Vatican and a version of Catholicism that embraced *caritas* over *agapé*, Martin Luther broke with the Church to form a new one: the Protestants. Once more, orthodox believers, like Old Testament Jews, quivered as sinners before an angry God who loved them despite their worthlessness. Encouraged by Savonarola, Luther set out to rid Christianity once and for all of any vestige of *eros*, Plato, and Aristotle.

Luther's attack on the Vatican also questioned the pope's claims to temporal authority. His message was compelling: Christians no longer needed a pope to mediate their relationship with God. By employing the more primitive *agapé* version of Christianity, one could commune directly with God and ask for His forgiveness themselves. This idea was revolutionary and resulted in Luther's breaking away from the Catholic Church and founding a new one, the Lutherans, the first Protestant religion, followed by a legion of others.

Though Luther saw his reforms as modest, they unleashed a plethora of competing Protestant religions, each claiming to possess the only true reading of the Bible. Among them was John Calvin, who argued that humans are worthless sinners whose fate was predestined by God even before they were born. Calvin advocated a return to the Old Testament God and delighted in depicting hellish tortures awaiting the vast majority of sinners in the afterlife, going beyond even Savonarola's fire and brimstone. Calvin's bleak vision spread throughout Great Britain, especially Scotland, and North America, generating capitalism, the rise of democracy, and entrepreneurship. Advocating a radical *agapé*-based notion of God's absolute control over one's fate, the thinking went that one might as well make hay while the sun shined and devote oneself to making as much money as possible, resulting in the so-called "Protestant work ethic." There is no better example of this spirit than the American evangelical right, driven by material wealth, worship of the stock market, and championing the likes of Donald Trump as their savior. This is an ironic consequence of the marginalization of the Catholic Church, which has always been associated with sexual repression.

Conclusion

What can we conclude from this brief exploration of *eros* and *agapé*? Despite the increasing secularization of modern culture in Europe, America seems just as Christianized as ever. Yet the Christian conception of *agapé*, characterized as distinct from *eros* as an inherently selfless love that accepts everyone, even one's enemies, blindly, is a fiction. *There is no such thing as selfless love.* All love, whatever name we give it, has *eros* as its foundation and is a tributary of it. This was Freud's great insight when he recognized that even *philia*, in the form of friendship, retains erotic elements. And thank God that it does! This is also the insight that both Augustine and Aquinas came to when they integrated *agapé* with *eros* by calling it *caritas*. They realized that all love contains pleasurable, erotic elements that were missing in Paul's conception of *agapé*. Paul's notion of love just wasn't real.

So what of the Christian argument that erotic love is egocentric and selfish and not fundamentally giving? We have just seen that the Christian conception of *agapé* is, ironically, *narcissistic*. It is even more egocentric than *eros* in the passive sense of the term. *Agapé* begins, first and foremost, with the love that God has for man, not with the love man has for God. It is inherently self-centered. The closest *agapé* comes to giving rather than taking love is by *imitating* God's love for man, as articulated in Thomas á Kempis's *Imitation of Christ* (2013). According to *agapé*, we don't need to do anything, be anybody, or perform any particular acts in order to win God's love. All we need do is pledge our allegiance to Him and embrace Him as our savior, and when we sin, which we are perfectly free to do as often as we wish, all that is required is to ask God's forgiveness, and it is granted. And what is our reward for doing absolutely nothing to deserve it? We die and go to Heaven for all eternity and enjoy endless and perpetual bliss. No wonder Christianity is the most popular religion in the world. What other religion would promise so much for giving up so little in return?

The impulse to give one's life to save another person, such as a child or a compatriot in battle, is rooted in *eros*, not *agapé*. This is what passion does to us. It makes us want to give. That is its essential impulse. Love of self and love of other comingle; neither is exclusive. This is why it also thrives on reciprocity, because we cannot love ourselves without someone to love in turn, someone who loves us too. All three – love of oneself, love for others, and feeling loved in return – are inseparable. You cannot single them out except in the abstract. That doesn't mean we love everyone the same, nor that we should. Some are more deserving of our love, and sometimes we too are less deserving than we might wish. This is why the ability to love, going back to Plato, is something we have to develop, in our own way, in our own time. *Eros* can also be destructive, selfish, vengeful, and insane. That too is in our nature. This holds true whether we are talking about love in a purely secular sense or whether we choose to imbue it with something divine.

So what can we learn from a conception of *agapé* that omits any reference to *eros*? That Freud was right. The most destructive force in human history is the repression of our most basic instinct: the desire to love passionately. This is why the principal purpose of psychoanalysis is to help undo the repressions we have accrued over a lifetime so that we may gradually, if painfully, become more loving. This not only leads to happiness. It makes us better human beings.

Notes

1   The Greeks emphasized *hubris* as the catalyst for *mania*, or madness. *Hubris* is unbridled desire, which compromises judgment and makes us irrational. The Greeks didn't seem to have a concept for neurosis. As conceptualized by Freud, neurosis is the consequence of *repressing* desire, not giving it free rein. This is a consequence of guilt, which is in turn the driving force of Christianity, whereas the Greeks lived in a shame-governed society, a society that is, perhaps, not as punitive as one's superego.

2   Following Plato, Freud recognized an erotic component to all love relationships, even the love of work, literature, and ideas. But instead of retaining Plato's terminology, Freud chooses to substitute "sexuality" in place of *Eros*, for reasons known only to Freud. The effect is nonetheless the same. Instead of the non-sexual edition, Freud opts for "non-genital" love, explaining that the explicitly sexual component is "aim-inhibited," as in friendships. This has brought Freud a lot of trouble, but he must have concluded it was preferable to stay with a common everyday word than to bring something Greek into the discussion. It wasn't exactly a secret, but Freud could be cagy about his sources and rarely invoked the Greeks when introducing his theories.

References

Aristotle (2000). *Nicomachean ethics* (Roger Crisp, Trans.). Cambridge: Cambridge University Press.

Kempis, Á. T. (2013). *The imitation of Christ*. Charlotte, NC: TAN Books.

Lewis, C. J. (2012). *The four loves: An exploration of the nature of love*. Boston and New York: Mariner Books, Houghton Mifflin Harcourt.

Plato (1991). *The symposium* (R. E. Allen, Trans.). New Haven and London: Yale University Press.

Chapter 11

The Biology of Love

Fritjof Capra, PhD

For the last 30 years I have developed a synthesis of a new conception of life, which is now emerging at the forefront of science. I call it "the systems view of life," which is also the title of the textbook I wrote with my colleague, Pier Luigi Luisi (Capra and Luisi, 2014). It is a synthesis that integrates four dimensions of life: the biological, the cognitive, the social, and the ecological.

In this work, I have occasionally come across natural scientists, like Humberto Maturana, who wrote about love. I have always shied away from using this word in my scientific work, but recently I have begun to see a connection between the human experience of love and the systems view of life. This was triggered by a German biologist and philosopher, Andreas Weber, who was a student of Francisco Varela and is therefore thoroughly familiar with the systems view of life. His book is titled *Matter and Desire* with the intriguing subtitle *An Erotic Ecology* (Weber, 2017). However, since *eros*, according to Plato, is desire in all its aspects, the link between Weber's two book titles, *Matter and Desire* and *An Erotic Ecology*, makes total sense. Indeed, the concept of love in the systems view of life, which I shall discuss in this essay, is related to the full dimension of *eros*, since it arises within a view of life that does not separate mind from body, reason from emotion, or human life from spirituality.

I shall first present a very brief summary of my synthesis of the systems view of life and then relate it to what Andreas Weber writes about love, life, and desire.

The Systems View of Life

In the systems view of life, the central characteristic of biological life is metabolism, defined as "the ceaseless flow of energy and matter through a network of chemical reactions, which enables a living organism to continually generate, repair, and perpetuate itself."

The understanding of metabolism includes two basic aspects. One is the continuous flow of energy and matter. All living systems need energy and food to sustain themselves, and all living systems produce waste. That's part of metabolism. But life has evolved in such a way that organisms form communities, the ecosystems, in which the waste of one species is food for the next, so that matter cycles continually through the ecosystem.

DOI: 10.4324/9781003564294-15

The second aspect of metabolism is the network of chemical reactions that process the food, and this forms the biochemical basis of all biological structures, functions, and behavior. The emphasis here is on "network." One of the most important insights of the systemic understanding of life is the recognition that networks are the basic pattern of organization of all living systems. Ecosystems are understood in terms of food webs (i.e., networks of organisms), organisms are networks of cells, and cells are networks of molecules. And then there are social systems, which are networks of communications. The network is a pattern that is common to all life. Wherever we see life, we see networks.

The defining characteristic of these living networks is that they are *self-generating*. In a cell, for example, all biological structures are continually produced, repaired, and regenerated by the cellular network. Similarly, at the level of a multicellular organism, the bodily cells are continually regenerated and recycled by the organism's metabolic network. Living networks continually create, or re-create, themselves by transforming or replacing their components. In this way they undergo continual structural changes while preserving their web-like patterns of organization. This coexistence of stability and change is indeed one of the key characteristics of life.

When we combine this insight with the one that no living organism can exist in isolation, that all organisms, to sustain themselves, need this continual flow of energy and matter, we realize that a living organism is engaged in continual interactions with its environment, each of which triggers structural changes in the system. This is why these interactions are known as "structural coupling." Living systems are autonomous, however. The environment only triggers the structural changes; it does not specify or direct them. A living system responds to a disturbance in its own, self-organizing way.

In the systems view of life, the process of this self-organizing response to disturbances is identified with cognition, the process of knowing. The interactions of a living organism – plant, animal, or human – with its environment are cognitive interactions. Thus, life and cognition are inseparably connected. The process of cognition – or, if you wish, of mind – is immanent in matter at all levels of life.

Now I have to come back to the flow aspect of metabolism. The dynamics of this flow of energy and matter through living networks have been studied in great detail and have led to a very important discovery. Living systems generally remain in a stable state, even though energy and matter flow through them and their structures are continually changing. But every now and then such an open system will encounter a point of instability where there is either a breakdown or, more frequently, a spontaneous emergence of new forms of order.

This spontaneous emergence of order at critical points of instability, which is often referred to simply as "emergence," is one of the hallmarks of life. It has been recognized as the dynamic origin of development, learning, and evolution. In other words, creativity – the generation of new forms – is a key property of all living systems.

And finally, I need to mention an important aspect of evolution. When we study the long history of evolution, we come to realize that nature sustains life by creating and nurturing communities. As soon as the first cells appeared on Earth, they formed tightly interlinked communities, known as bacterial colonies, and for billions of years, nature has maintained such communities at all levels of life. Life flourishes in communities, in networks of relationships.

Human Experience of the Characteristics of Life

These are the main concepts of the systems view of life: the description of living systems in terms of networks and flows; the continual self-generation and regeneration of these living networks; the ongoing interactions of living organisms with their environment, while they maintain their autonomy; cognition as the dynamics of self-organization, as the very process of life; the spontaneous emergence of order – in other words, life's inherent creativity; and the flourishing of life in communities, in networks of relationships.

These phenomena are characteristic of all forms of life, from the simplest bacteria and other microorganisms, to plants, animals, and human beings. We can experience them at the human level, and when the fundamental characteristics of life are experienced by a conscious self, they acquire new meaning.

For example, we experience the autonomy of our living organism as free will; the emergence of new ideas or new artistic forms as human creativity; the processes of relationships with others as animosity, affection, or love; and behavior for the common good as ethical behavior. To attribute these human values and emotions to other forms of life would be anthropomorphism, but we must realize that they are based on biological patterns and processes common to all life.

Love as a Longing for Attachment

I have now prepared the ground to discuss some of Andreas Weber's key ideas. His starting point is the observation that life flourishes in communities, in networks of relationships. In fact, an individual self can be seen as a node in a network of relationships. Who I am depends on my personal and professional relationships to others, on my relationships to ideas and cultural traditions, as well as on the genetic relationships to my ancestors. Weber writes:

> We long to connect with another – be it world, skin, food, or air – in order to become ourselves.
>
> (Weber, 2017, p. xiv)

He identifies this longing for connecting with another with the biological basis of love:

> In all living systems, the drive, desire, and longing for attachment *and* autonomy is foundational: essential in order to perceive, to continue, and to unfold.
>
> (p. xiii)

Now, I would argue with Weber's use of "desire" and "longing" to describe this drive for attachment in simple organisms. In my view, living organisms (at least before the emergence of emotions in evolution) don't "long to connect" – they just connect. Only at higher levels of consciousness, which involve the ability to create mental images and to imagine the future, can there be desire. However, to ground the human experience of love in this biological reality seems a valid idea to me.

Erotic Ecology

The next step for Weber is to note that ecology is essentially a science of relationships. "This book," he writes, "describes ecological reality as a relational system. And conversely, it comprehends love as an ecological process" (p. xiv). The fundamental experience of these ecological relationships, for him, is the experience of being touched, which is an erotic experience; thus, his term "an erotic ecology." Here are a few more passages:

> Being in the world is primarily an erotic encounter, an encounter of meaning through contact, an encounter of being oneself through the significance of others.
>
> (xiii)

> From birth, and probably even before it, we experience the fundamental erotics of being touched by the world.
>
> (p. xiv)

This is, of course, very Freudian. According to Freud, the desire to be touched is our strongest desire. Touch, in Freud's view, is the very essence of *eros*. Trauma is the disruption of touch, and because touch is essential to life, the disruption of touch becomes a disruption of life, and hence an existential problem. Most psychiatrists search for the "causes" of trauma, which can then be counteracted. Freud, by contrast, saw neurosis as a creative response to certain life situations, and Laing had the same understanding of psychosis.

Another interesting idea is that, according to Laing, "psychotherapy, essentially, is an authentic meeting between human beings" (quoted in Capra, 1988, p. 115). In my view, this was the essence of his approach. In his authentic encounters with patients, Laing touched them deeply. They felt "touched" or "moved," and through this metaphorical touching he helped them to overcome their traumas, to "metabolize" them, as it were.

Now back to Andreas Weber. I found it interesting how he relates erotic touch to the concept of structural coupling (the interactions of a living system with its environment, which trigger structural changes in the system). He writes:

> We discern the fundamental principles of erotic touch: two sides always enter into relationship such that both come away changed.
>
> (p. 22)

The world is not an aggregation of things, but rather a symphony of relationships between many participants that are altered by the interaction: a necessarily erotic occurrence.

(p. 29)

Love as Aliveness

The biological and ecological phenomena Weber associates with love – the network of relationships, the individual as a node in such a network, and the structural changes triggered by each interaction – are all fundamental characteristics of life, and so he comes to the conclusion that, ultimately, the experience of love is an experience of intense aliveness:

I have the impression that love is nothing more or less than pure aliveness in flesh and blood. . . . To love means to be fully alive.

(p. 3)

It is interesting that the feeling of intense aliveness has also been associated with spiritual experience. To begin with, the original meaning of spirit is "breath." Spirit is the breath of life. The Benedictine monk, psychologist, and author David Steindl-Rast characterizes spiritual experience as moments of heightened aliveness (Steindl-Rast, 1990). Our spiritual moments, according to Brother David, are those moments when we feel most intensely alive. The aliveness felt during such a "peak experience," as Abraham Maslow called it, involves not only the body but also the mind.

Buddhists refer to this heightened mental alertness as "mindfulness," and they emphasize that mindfulness is deeply rooted in the body. Spirituality, then, is always embodied. Spiritual experience is an experience of aliveness of mind and body as a unity. Moreover, this experience of unity transcends not only the separation of mind and body, but also the separation of self and world. The central awareness in these spiritual moments is a profound sense of oneness with all, a sense of belonging to the universe a whole. And of course, as we all know, love too involves the dissolution of ego boundaries.

So, here we have spirituality characterized by an intense sense of aliveness and by a sense of fundamental connectedness – exactly as in Andreas Weber's understanding of love. What is missing in Brother David's description of spiritual experience is the sense of longing and the erotic touch. But if you read the writings of mystics, like Saint Teresa of Avila, or look at paintings and sculptures of saints in ecstasy, there is plenty of longing and erotic intensity.

Desire as a Life Wish

Living organisms maintain themselves in a delicate coexistence of stability and change. Whenever they reach a point of instability, there can be a spontaneous emergence of novelty, or a breakdown of the system. According to Weber,

A life-form can fail at any time, and therefore it *wants* to survive.

[Desire is] the wish for continued existence. . . . The life wish is not a program, but an urge that emerges out of matter and also structures it. A being –
even the simplest cell – *is* this longing.

(pp. 43–44)

Again, I am not comfortable with this formulation from the scientific point of view,
even though I like it as poetry. As a scientist, I would simply say that in evolution,
those organisms that organize themselves to assure their continued existence are
the ones that survive. I don't see the need to project longing or desire onto them.

Metabolism and Death

All living systems sustain their continued existence through metabolism. As I have
mentioned, metabolism is the ceaseless flow of energy and matter through a network of chemical reactions, which enables a living organism to continually generate, repair, and perpetuate itself. Metabolism involves the continual creation and
transformation of components. In the case of a multicellular organism, it involves
the continual regeneration and recycling of cells. This constant recycling of cells
is part of the organism's self-renewal, which is an essential property of life. But
what is self-renewal at the level of the organism is the cycle of life and death at the
level of the recycled cells. In other words, the death of an individual cell is not the
opposite of life, but is an essential aspect of life at a higher systems level.

Andreas Weber writes a lot about this important connection between metabolism, the essence of life, and death. Here is what he writes about metabolism:

In contrast to an object or machine, a body regularly splits off a part of itself in
order to survive and incorporates a piece of the foreign world into itself. This
is precisely why it is wrong to compare a life-form with a machine: a machine
does not metabolize.

(p. 57)

Cells can only survive by casting off their substance and building themselves
anew in every moment out of the flesh of other beings.

(p. 67)

The functioning of the circle of life on Earth depends solely on the fact that we
all share in the great body of matter and pass through one another reciprocally.

(p. 57)

Now, I have also written a lot about metabolism, but never in such a poetic way,
and this time I completely agree with what he says. And here he is on life and death:

Aliveness must be able to fail, if it is truly alive. Only because of death does life
become creative.

(p. 50)

While in the prime of life, every cell is dying a continual death.

(p. 56)

Death is the way in which the living make an offering so that more life emerges.

(p. 197)

And finally, here is an interesting observation about the failure of most cultures to understand this essential link between life and death:

The central misery of all cultures (not just ours) is the denial brought about by our permanent fear of death. . . . People of all eras have striven for immortality by various means: the worship of omnipresent ancestors in rocks and trees, the eternal life that awaits all true believers, the technological deliverance that will allow the world to be conquered. There has always been a heroic path to immortality. Following this path has always required strict rules that required one to give up the very thing that was supposed to be preserved: one's own aliveness.

(p. 153)

References

Capra, F. (1988). *Uncommon wisdom*. New York: Simon and Schuster.

Capra, F. and Luisi, P. L. (2014). *The systems view of life*. New York: Cambridge University Press.

Steindl-Rast, D. (1990). Spirituality as common sense. *The Quest*, 3, no. 2.

Weber, A. (2017). *Matter and desire*. White River Junction, VT: Chelsea Green.

Chapter 12

Laing on Love

Douglas Kirsner, PhD

Love lies at the heart of Laing's general approach. This chapter will sketch out the basic approach and parameters that Laing adopted, sourcing his works, films, interviews and lectures he delivered in the 1960s and 1970s.

For Laing, love is central to the study of human beings. It cannot be excluded without grossly distorting the method and what is observed and understood. According to Laing, 'Love reveals facts which, without it, remain undisclosed' (Laing, 1976a, p. 97).

Thus, Laing was very concerned about the factoring out of love in the acquisition, description and evaluation of knowledge that brings about a false objectivity that feeds on itself, appearing to exclude human intention and action as major factors. Knowledge about human beings should, of necessity, factor in human values, contributions and involvements. It needs to be personal. The final page of Laing's memoir to his age of 30, *Wisdom, Madness and Folly* (1985), is about the exclusion of the personal from psychiatry. The personal, Laing avers, is ignored and feared by professionals as much as it is by patients.

'Psychiatry', Laing declares, 'tries to be as scientific, impersonal and objective as possible towards what is most personal and subjective'. According to Laing, psychiatric treatment concerns our innermost personal thoughts and desires. Western medical training does nothing to equip doctors to integrate the personal with clinical work. So, in the face of inner suffering, doctors become disoriented given their conventional training (Laing, 1985, p. 146).

Having written *The Divided Self*, by the age of 30, Laing says, he knew he wanted to address himself to 'integrating the personal factor in theory and practice' (Laing, 1985 p. 146). The personal along with the exclusion of the personal are abiding and dominant themes throughout Laing's future work. No other term has been more prostituted than love and its exclusion (Laing, 1965a, p. 34).

As Laing states in *The Divided Self*, a science deals with what is appropriate to its field, and the study of human beings entails the human prisms to see what is going on. As he suggests in *The Divided Self*, the appropriate science for human beings is the science of persons. Diagnosis, for Laing, is etymologically 'seeing through', which involved both *seeing* through the prism of what goes on as much as seeing *through* to the reality of what is going on. By valuing what we *see*, we can

DOI: 10.4324/9781003564294-16

ignore what we see *through*. The human context is ineradicable even if its elimination may appear more attractive to a scientific, objectivist approach of modern times. The more intention and love are factored out of the equation, the more they appear irrelevant. Yet that exclusion distorts the phenomenological context still further.

Love is and has always been a many-splendored thing, which needs to be seen in the context of the use of the term. Just as Eskimos have many terms for snow, the Greeks who studied love had, as Michael Thompson has found, at least eight terms for love. So we have *eros*, erotic love; *caritas*, charitable love; *agape*, or spiritual love; and *philia*, or filial love. Love was so central to Laing that he, with some colleagues, founded the Philadelphia Association in 1965 with filial love as its guiding principle. It was set up as a charity to utilize an open-minded alternative approach to mental illness and psychotherapy on the basis of *philia*, or brotherly or sisterly love. The brochure from the early period declared on its frontispiece:

Philadelphia (Greek): brotherly or sisterly love. '. . . I have set before thee an open door, and no man can shut it'.

(Revelation 3.8)

The articles of association include these aims:

To relieve mental illness of all descriptions, in particular schizophrenia.
To undertake, and further, research into the causes of mental illness, the means of its detection and prevention, and its treatment.
To provide, and further, the profusion of residential accommodation for persons suffering or who have suffered from mental illness. (Philadelphia Association brochure)

The Philadelphia Association, based as it was upon love, became a central thread in Laing's life and work.

Aristotle's modes of friendship significantly include love in terms of three approaches – love as about utility or business, achieving useful aims; love as providing pleasure or entertainment; and what we often think of as true love, the love that values the other in terms of his or her true nature, or is-ness, as valuable for its own sake. *Eros* plays a central part in Freud's approach both in its general sense of life energy and in its decisive role in many kinds of relationships. And who can forget the pleasure principle? Although the term 'love' is used across a range of contexts with many meanings and aspects, love always involves something distinctively human. We exclude love as a crucial factor at the peril of losing any real understanding of our fundamental mode of being.

From the eighteenth-century onwards, objectivity became the lynchpin of the scientific conception of the nature of knowledge itself. Being objective is valued in the natural sciences over subjective, and subjectivity is seen as best eliminated in science. This has both positive and negative aspects. On the positive side, the scientific and technological world of modern human beings has brought about massive advances in our quantity and quality of life. The overarching natural scientific approach and look ought not be condemned in a blanket way. As Laing says, he wants the dentist to take a scientific and detached look at his teeth and how best to treat them (Kirsner, 2013, p. 367). This involves context and the appropriate and nuanced use of science and technology as a most useful servant, but not master, for human ends. There has been an overextension of science into aspects of human existence where it is not appropriate to apply, such as the choice of human ends, decisions and understanding our inner and interpersonal experiential worlds. As Pascal put it, 'The heart has its reasons that reason does not know'. Psychoanalysis, which focuses on experience, was formed in that era too. But by and large, natural science involves trying not to tamper with the observations by taking the person out of the equation, especially when it comes to human issues.

Laing says that contemporary science is characterizable by a phrase of C. F. von Weizsacker, a twentieth-century German theoretical physicist and philosopher, who declared, when summarizing the nature of modern science,

> The scientific and technical world of modern man is a result of his daring enterprise: knowledge without love. The serpent in paradise urges on man knowledge without love. Antichrist is the power in the history that leads loveless knowledge into the battle of destruction against love. But it is at the same time the power that destroys itself in its triumph. The battle is still raging. We are in the midst of it, at a post not of our choosing, where we must prove ourselves.
>
> (von Weizsäcker, 1949, p. 190)

A major problem lies in the mindset of scientists and doctors who have often been trained to dissect frogs and cut up dead animals, taking them apart to see how they move. What is the relationship between dissecting a frog and talking to a psychotic? This training distances the doctor and scientist from life, moving on and generalizing from dissecting animals to understanding the meaning and purposes of human beings.

If we aim to understand or know one another better, Laing says it makes a difference if such knowledge is based upon whether love is excluded from the intentions or objects of study. You can only recognize the existence of love by being open to its being there (Laing, 1975). Laing suggests that feeling for others means 'that one leaves the other alone, that one in fact doesn't interfere, influence, tamper with, or in any way transgress or intrude grossly or subtly on the being of the other person'. He recalls that St. Thomas Aquinas even defines love as the knowledge of being in itself, in its is-ness. Without the presence of love, many human facts remain undisclosed (see Laing, 1976a, p. 97). Laing explains that we can't know what our essential being is if one tampers with it – like trying to make ice by boiling water. As the Tao Te Ching says, 'Those that tamper with it harm it. Those that grab it lose it'. Without a feeling for the other, one unknowingly tramples on them (Laing, 1976a, p. 97).

Thus, Laing was concerned with love as not being tampered with so that the other is left to be who they are. This certainly resonates with Buddhist concepts of attachment and detachment. In any case, we can see that the observer is part of the observational field and affects what is observed. How we approach the other affects what we see, and whether the approach is with or without love in the equation makes all the difference.

A chapter in *The Politics of Experience*, 'The Mystification of Experience', originally titled 'Violence and Love' (Laing, 1965b), contains insights in terms of understanding and updating Karl Marx's original concept of mystification, which is helpful to understanding Laing's contributions to the nature of therapy. Whatever its rhetorical attributes, 'Violence and Love' demonstrates an unusual lack of nuance on Laing's part. Although individual detail and nuance are normally an essential part of Laing's skeptical approach, the chapter is more a poetic and rhetorical desperate plea, akin to Alan Ginsberg's *Howl*. Laing adapts Marx's concept of 'mystification' to add the forms of reciprocal interaction of person with person to the psychological realm. Marx uses the idea of mystification to explain what happens when social relations are obscured or how far social relations form the world (see Chapter 5).

For Laing, individuals are not islands, and interactions and perceptions mold behavior and judgment of experience. Laing suspects that there may be different interactions within families, especially those with schizophrenic members. Laing understood the nature of our inevitable interactions as involving communication, ascription and commands that needed decrypting or deciphering.

Love is a prime vehicle for mystification in Laing's view. During the mid-1960s, Laing views love through the prism of overwhelming and ubiquitous violence that so often masquerades as love. He proposes then that human beings are violated to the core in modern times, that we are influenced and manipulated at every level, beyond our knowing just like Herbert Marcuse's one-dimensional man (see Marcuse, 1964). Since violence seems to inhabit every aspect of the contemporary world even down to the devastation of experience, there is no room for love as such to even begin. Laing's *The Politics of the Family* (1971) is a critique of the family demonstrating the destruction that goes on in the most intimate relationships, principally through mystification and confusion.

Freud is acutely aware of the disturbances to love that come with culture or civilization. During a 1980 interview with me, Laing refers to Freud's comment in *Civilization and Its Discontents* where Freud stated:

Among the works of the sensitive English writer, John Galsworthy . . . there is a short story of which I early formed a high opinion. It is called 'The Apple-Tree': and it brings home to us how the life of present- day civilized people leaves no room for the simple natural love of two human beings.

(Freud, 1930 [1961], p. 105)

Writing around the same period as he wrote 'Violence and Love', Laing declares in his 1964 Preface to the Pelican Edition of *The Divided Self*:

> Freud insisted that our civilization is a repressive one. There is a conflict between the demands of conformity and the demands of our instinctive energies, explicitly sexual. Freud could see no easy resolution of this antagonism, and he came to believe that in our time the possibility of simple natural love between human beings had already been abolished.
>
> (Laing, 1965a, p. 10)

Perhaps *The Politics of Experience* is also in part Laing's update of *Civilization and Its Discontents*. Love is inevitably tampered with by society so that there is no way it can emerge. Laing suggests:

> Love and violence, properly speaking, are polar opposites. Love lets the other be, but with affection and concern. Violence attempts to constrain the other's freedom, to force him to act in the way we desire, but with ultimate lack of concern, with indifference to the other's own existence or destiny.
>
> (Laing, 1967a, p. 50)

This is all part of the fundamental error of treating persons as things or objects to be manipulated. According to Laing, persons experience, whereas things behave. The natural scientific method that doesn't recognize this ends up with reified results and doesn't recognize the fundamental

> ontological discontinuity between human beings and it-beings. Human beings relate to each other not simply externally, like two billiard balls, but by the relations of the two worlds of experience that come into play when two people meet. If human beings are not studied as human beings, then this once more is violence and mystification.
>
> (Laing, 1967, p. 53)

For Laing in 1965, violence and intrusion were so ubiquitous, everything was so tampered, with that there was no room for love, which is on that account necessarily a fraud and a swindle. Laing certainly modified his position on love as he abandoned the all-encompassing, overarching, simplistic political view, and also as he found love himself personally.

But all along, the principle of the idea of love itself is crucial to his philosophy and sensibility. As I suggested in Chapter 2, Laing was a classical liberal or libertarian on the model of John Stuart Mill. He begins from the individual and their freedom of choice, not from the collective. His model of 'live and let live' is about leaving the individual alone within the law to pursue their own goals in their own way. Laing agrees with both Sartre and Mill that the ability of the individual to make their own choices is a good in itself. Not being intruded upon, being left alone to be as free as possible to develop in one's own way, not being tampered with or violated even for one's own alleged good, instead but respected, nurtured, cared for or nurtured so that one can blossom in one's own way lies at the heart of Laing's approach across the board, including to human relations, psychiatry, therapy, politics, society, science and technology, birth, spirituality and love.

But then, what is the nature of that love, and is it possible in practice?

From early in his life Laing was acutely aware of issues that stand in the way of love from an early age, some of which are so obvious that they are hard to see. He recalls in *Did You Used to Be R. D. Laing* (1989):

I can remember vividly around the age of 7 or 8 a boy in my class at school. I went to his house, another house, another world, amazing. I think that type of childhood I had has obviously sensitized me to this area of life more than most other people are sensitized to this area. So it occasions me maybe the greatest consolations I've had in life. And the greatest pain I've had in life have been in relationship to other people.

Laing continues speaking with the song 'Nobody Knows the Trouble I've Seen' in the background on the film:

From my earliest days in Glasgow, Scotland where I was born in 1927, there was my father and mother, and they did they did not seem to be happy. And I addressed myself at that time to why did these people seem to be so miserable, what are they unhappy about? It had a great deal to do with how they were not getting on very well with each other. And they were entangled, and I was entangled. And they were entangled with all those terribly little things that I have spent the last 50 of my 60 years or so since I was about 10 years old trying to figure out. A lot of it seems to go around the issue of love.

Laing's own early bad personal experience of love continued in one way or another into the early and mid-1960s, when he was very negative about the real chances of love. But then he met Jutta, a resident of Kingsley Hall, during 1966 and 1967, and love bloomed. They married in 1974 and had two sons and a daughter together. There was a bad breakup when Jutta left him, then divorced him in 1988. Some of this in a fictionalized way is portrayed in the film, *Mad to Be Normal* (Mullan, 2017). So it is interesting to trace the evolution of Laing's views on love in tandem with his own experiences from childhood to some miserable years, good years, and then some miserable ones again.

Much of Laing's project is to explain why this is the case by deconstructing the knots, ties, tangles, impasses and deceptions that challenge or even may masquerade as love, that stand in the way of the fruition of love. He doesn't question love as such, but the obstacles to love; sometimes even the possibility of love. He maps how violent behavior may appear to be love or even masquerade as love. Treating people without respect or labeling them might appear to everybody involved to be in their own best interests.

But the obstacles to love may not be deliberately created. The term 'masquerading' sounds intentionally deceptive, but it may not be. Laing was captivated by investigations into communications and interpersonal perceptions, how we don't know what each other thinks and certainly not whether they know that we know what they do or that we know what they think we think we think they think. People may be deceived that they are not deceived. We are often mystified and confused in our perceptions and intentions, and Laing wanted to see how the knots in the politics of relationships could be untangled, how the codes could be deciphered. Laing remarked in a lecture to the White Institute in 1967 that Freud's classic work, *The Psychopathology of Everyday Life*, is about 'how the truth will out'. And this may often be unbeknown to ourselves at the time, such as in slips of the tongue or jokes.

Laing asks, 'Do you love me? Nobody loves you. . . . Believe me, . . . Don't believe me but don't believe me because I say so. That's my mother', Laing recalls of his mother whom he regarded as a witch, an understandable charge, given that she made a voodoo doll of him and used to stick pins into it at night. Laing was tortured by love all his life, obsessed with love and how destructive families can be. Laing felt many people got caught in this kind of trap that 'they ought to trust or believe the person they love because they love them' (Laing, 1989).

But Laing didn't see why that would follow, given that we are used to so much disinformation, even fake news, and deception everywhere. This is even more true in relation to sexual relationships. But Laing claims, 'Bedrooms are the most dangerous places on God's earth. They are more dangerous than the streets of Los Angeles. More crimes of violence are committed in bedrooms. More murders are committed in bedrooms than in any other location' (Laing, 1989). Laing was clearly seized by the need to be clear-sighted as to what is actually taking place so as to act meaningfully. Unknotting the tangles that love has woven along with everything else is essential in this. According to Laing,

> Any illusion, any idealization, any disparagement, any way we have of projecting, or denying the existence of the other person as he or she is in his or her own is-ness is not loving them. Really to be with another person in a completely open-hearted unguarded way where one is not on one's own part canceling or changing or altering or modifying who that other person is to suit one's own book.
>
> (Laing, 1989)

Laing contrasts this with co-presence, which is being actually present to each other without reservation, a precondition to communion, which he thought the perfect way we should ordinarily be together.

In *The Facts of Life*, Laing describes how a patient came downstairs at home to see her husband with a naked woman. Thereupon her husband told her, 'That isn't a woman, that is a waterfall'. And she felt she was spinning around she might faint. . . . Some people in that moment of vertigo lose themselves by believing what they're told at the expense of then you can't believe your eyes or believe your ears', Laing explains. This is not the same as jealousy, but in addition to the pain of discovery of having been deceived and betrayed, one's sense of reality is blown and may lead to having to revise one's entire history. I remember Laing telling the story of an elderly patient who had just discovered that her husband had a mistress – for 40 years! She came to Laing not because of jealousy, but primarily because her whole history and sense of reality lay in tatters. According to Laing, 'I am sure that truth deprivation can wreak as much havoc in some people as vitamin deprivation' (Laing, 1976a, p. 145). Believing or not believing your eyes has ontological consequences. Derealization, the sense of reality breaking down, betrayal and deep ontological insecurity can contribute to driving a person crazy.

Laing was greatly influenced by Jean-Paul Sartre's dark views on human relations, from Sartre's early to late works, which always focused on how almost invariably tangled up relationships are, even with the best of intentions. For Sartre, relationships are always conflict-ridden wrestles for control in a master-slave dialectic and are locked in conflict as either sadistic or masochistic. *Do You Love Me?* could be a remake of Sartre's 1944 play, *No Exit*, where 'Hell is other people'. Sartre's later work, which Laing approved of, focuses on the oppressive structures of groups where outcomes so often resulted in counter-finality, that is, the opposite of what was intended in a game of Loser Wins. Laing was intent on revealing the games people play, often unbeknown to themselves or even others. 'Games People Play' was a Grammy Award song debuted by Joe South in 1968 and covered by Jerry Lee Lewis, Tina Turner and Inner Circle, among others.

A too often neglected book on the dynamics of communication and miscommunication, *Interpersonal Perception* (Laing et al., 1966), researched the differences between levels of communication – questioning what I think, what I think you think, what I think you think I think, and so on. This is along with what you think, what you think I think, what you think I think you think, etc., and how these all meld or mostly don't meld together. I often attribute my own perceptions to others, and vice versa, so that systematic miscommunications occur. Then there are the repressions, invalidation beyond confusions, misattributions and projections that result in mystifications and reifications. It's a matter of levels of communication, sometimes confused and conflicting with each other. So a communication on one level might clash with a communication on a meta level, without conscious awareness. This was the double bind or double message that could drive people crazy – well known in the work of Gregory Bateson and Harold Searles – come here and go away at the same time. Or a message of 'I love you' while simultaneously communicating pushing in the opposite direction on a non-verbal level. So, it is a political kind of challenge in communications to try to reveal and unshackle mystifications, confusions and conflicts within dyadic and group family structures. Laing moved beyond a one-person psychology to at least a two-person psychology or even a group systemic psychology. Laing saw the big innovations of the 1960s as the revolution in understanding the science of communications. Love is the perfect storm location for different levels of communications, given the physical, neurological, mental, spiritual, linguistic, non-verbal, irrational, unconscious, passionate and intense levels of communication involved. Moreover, Laing was seriously focused on understanding game theory or set theory in terms of group theory and transformations involving mapping from one set onto another. Thus, there is an overlay or imprint from one generation only to another in a transference over space and time. People today are influenced by the image of their parents and grandparents from the past, with projections and introjections that remain active.

However, the clash, conflict and interplay of levels are what is particularly confusing and mystifying from Laing's perspective. He begins *Knots* with this simple form:

> They are playing a game. They are playing at not playing a game. If I show them I think they are, I will break the rules and they will punish me.
> I must play their game, of not seeing I see the game.

(Laing, 1970, p. 1)

Here is one example from *Knots* of the form of interpersonal misperceptions that are way beyond a one-person psychology that can stand in the way of harmony in a relationship:

> Jack can see that he sees
> what Jill can't see
> but Jack can't see
> that Jill can't see
> that Jill can't see it.
>
> Jack tries to get Jill to see
> that Jack can see
> what Jill can't see
> but Jack can't see
> that Jill can't see that Jill can't see it.
>
> Jack sees
> there is something Jill can't see
> and Jack sees
> that Jill can't see she can't see it.
>
> Although Jack can see Jill can't see she can't see it
> he can't see that he can't see it himself (Laing, 1970, p. 57).

Here is a similar dynamic from *Do You Love Me?* that questions and reveals some of the patterns of the obstacles in love's path:

> **Do you love me?**
>
> do you love me?
> yes I love you

best of all?
yes best of all
more than the whole world?
yes more than the whole world
do you like me
yes I like you
do you like being near me?
yes I like being near you . . .

do you really love me?
yes I really love you
say "I love you"
I love you
do you want to hug me?

yes I want to hug you, and cuddle you
and bill and coo with you . . .
swear you'll never leave me
I swear I'll never ever leave you, cross my heart
and hope to die if I tell a lie
(*pause*)
do you *really* love me? (Laing, 1976b, pp. 85–86)

What does all this have to do with therapy? A great deal, since it reveals how therapy can heal by not tampering with people, being empathic and there with them and valuing and respecting their subjectivity. Laing himself had the uncanny ability to bring love out in the most existential sense of letting the other be in their own space and way, not manipulate or change them, but get to know them. A kind of love and nurturing. The further means of doing so is to explore distortions, tangles, knots, impasses, mystifications and confusions to recognize what is going on and help bring about more trust and ontological security in oneself and close others if possible. Love is not intrinsically destructive, or else therapy would be impossible.

References

Freud, S. (1930[1961]). Civilization and its discontents. In J. Strachey (ed.), *The future of an illusion, civilization and its discontents, and other works. The standard edition of the complete psychological works of Sigmund Freud*, Vol. 21, pp. 64–145 (1927–1931). London: Hogarth Press and the Institute of Psychoanalysis.

Kirsner, D. (2013). Human, all too human: Interview with R. D. Laing. *Psychoanalytic Review*, 100, no. 2: 361–372.

Laing, R. D. (1965a). *The divided self: An existential study in sanity and madness*. Harmondsworth: Penguin Books.

Laing, R. D. (1965b). Mystification, confusion and conflict. In I. Boszormenyi-Nagy and J. L. Framo (eds.), *Intensive family therapy*, pp. 343–363. New York: Harper and Row.

Laing, R. D. (1967a). Family and social contexts in relation to the origin of schizophrenia. In J. Romano (ed.), *Proceedings of the First Rochester international conference on schizophrenia*, March 29–31, 1967, *Excerpta Medica*, International Conference Series, 151, Amsterdam, pp. 139–145.

Laing, R. D. (1967b). *The politics of experience and the bird of paradise*. Harmondsworrth: Penguin Books.

Laing, R. D. (1970). *Knots*. New York: Pantheon.

Laing, R. D. (1971). *The politics of the family and other essays*. London: Tavistock.

Laing, R. D. (1975). What is the Philadelphia Association? *Lecture*, November 12. Unpublished.

Laing, R. D. (1976a). *The facts of life*. London: Allen Lane.

Laing, R. D. (1976b). *Do you love me? An entertainment in conversation and verse*. New York: Pantheon.

Laing, R. D. (1985). *Wisdom, madness and folly: The making of a psychiatrist*. London: Macmillan.

Laing, R. D. (1989). *Did you used to be R. D. Laing?* TV Movie. Third Mind Productions, Channel 4 Films, TVO, Canada, UK.

Laing, R. D., Phillipson, H., and Lee, A. R. (1966). *Interpersonal perception: A theory and a method of research*. Oxford: Springer.

Marcuse, H. (1964). *One-dimensional man: Studies in ideology of advanced industrial society*. Boston: Beacon Press.

Mullan, R. (2017). *Mad to be normal*. Gizmo Films–Bad Penny Productions. UK.

von Weizsäcker, C. F. (1949). *The history of nature*. Chicago: University of Chicago Press.

V

What Is Authenticity?

Chapter 13

Laing on Authenticity

Douglas Kirsner, PhD

How can we be authentic in a world we don't choose? How can we be true to ourselves if there is no essential self to be true to? How can we go beyond our false selves? Laing, following Jean-Paul Sartre, responds to such conundrums by unmasking, mapping and revealing patterns of self-deception, deceptions and false-self systems in individual and social contexts.

Laing's approach was fundamentally existentialist in nature, as Laing was no utilitarian and placed fundamental value on the uniqueness of the individual and their experience. From Laing's perspective, authenticity is good in itself and is intrinsically valuable and is not good because it has better consequences, even if it does. Maxims such as 'Know thyself' and 'An unexamined life is not worth living' reflect foundational ethical values that underline an existentialist approach to human realities built upon individual freedom, choice and responsibility rather than the consequentialism of the hedonic balances of pleasure and pain. I am sure he would have agreed with John Stuart Mill's famous statement, 'It is better to be a human being dissatisfied than a pig satisfied; better to be Socrates dissatisfied than a fool satisfied' (Mill, 1863, Chapter 2).

Thus it's curious that in spite of the fact that the concept of authenticity pervades Laing's life and writings from *The Divided Self* onwards, Laing didn't often use the term 'authenticity'. For Laing, authenticity is not so much a direct striving for personal truth as about revealing how we avoid the obvious, that which stands in front of us, by mystifyingly constructing false selves and false-self systems so as not to see what is going on.

Laing was an anti-systematic thinker who focused less on finding the right answers than on asking the right questions. He didn't want to account for the content of a true self so much as understand how we erect barriers to avoid our freedom. Throughout, Laing is interested in revealing and deciphering the false-self systems that stand in the way of our being real.

Laing's view of authenticity owed much to the legacy of existentialism. He adopted the ideas of Heidegger and Sartre about the foundation of the irreducible freedom that constitutes us. We construct our lives and meaning with no essential self, but rather as active self as agent. The focus is not on the nature and content of

DOI: 10.4324/9781003564294-18

a true self, but upon how we construct false selves and illusion and how we might be able to map and go beyond them.

Such a long-standing, difficult and frustrating journey is reflected in this story from the Talmud:

A man once got lost in the thick of the forest. For days he tried hopelessly to find his way out, yet it was to no avail. This continued for many weeks and months. One day, he came across an old man, who was coming toward him. He ran to the stranger and pleaded, 'Please tell me how to get out of this forest – I have been wandering for many weeks and months!'

'My son', the old man replied forlornly, 'unfortunately, I too am lost. I have been wandering in this forest not for weeks nor months, but for many years, yet I still have not found the way out. However, before you conclude that any advice I may offer is certainly useless, consider this: Although I may not know the way out of the forest, I can tell you better than anyone which paths lead to nowhere!'

(Torah.com 2024 https://torah.org/torah-portion/
olas-shabbos-5761-behaaloscha/)

I think that Laing was mapping the obstacles and the paths that don't work rather than directly showing the way out.

The term 'authenticity' had a bad press in the 1970s when it often appeared, ironically, to be fake, not genuine, people playing at or pretending to themselves and others to be authentic. People could tell themselves they were who they wished to be instead of who they really were. Wishing, hoping, pretending instead of recognizing reality and moving on from there sound, in fact, more authentic.

It was often a buzz word, adopting the empty language of self-centered self-absorption aiming to express the subdued inner child of pop psychology.

But is there something beyond this?

The original meaning of being authentic ('to thine own self be true') is what something really, purely or genuinely is. As Sartre would have it, authenticity implies being true to one's own set of commitments. This builds upon Jean-Jacques Rousseau's 18th-century paradox that we are born free but are everywhere in chains. For Rousseau, the introduction of private property corrupted the purity of children. Although Rousseau's view is based upon a simplistic view of an essentially good self of 'noble savages', it serves also to call into question established, taken-for-granted social hierarchical assumptions.

Laing immersed himself in reading the existentialists in his early years. For Laing, Sartre was a 'gate-opener to the tradition that Sartre espoused, Hegel, Husserl, Heidegger' (Charlesworth, 1973, p. 49). Laing read Sartre's *Being and Nothingness* (1943[1984]), which built upon many of Heidegger's concepts before he read Heidegger's earlier classic, *Being and Time* (Heidegger, 1927[1962]).

Although the concept of 'authenticity' used in existential philosophy originated with Kierkegaard's book, *Sickness unto Death*, it was expounded classically in Heidegger's *Being and Time*. Heidegger actually coined the term *Eigentlichkeit*, translated early as 'authenticity', from the ordinary German word *Eisgentlich*, meaning 'actually', 'truly' or 'really', which built upon the German word *Eigen*, meaning own or proper. For Heidegger, authenticity involves owning up to who we are or being one's own, the quality of ownedness – dis-owning it is inauthentic. For Heidegger, the noise of the world covers up and distracts us from the uncanniness of our being-in-the-world. Recognizing this uncanniness allows us to further experience our 'fallenness' and ourselves as 'thrown' in our essential estrangement. Thus, a sense of estrangement or alienation from others, for Heidegger, is a good thing, not a bad thing, because it represents a basis for becoming attuned to our authentic mode of being rather than being absorbed into the world of the 'they' or others. In Heidegger's account, to be uniquely human involves our agency whereby we shape our identity, realizing our individual human distinctiveness through owning and realizing our overarching projects for the sake of ourselves.

Heidegger, who built upon Nietzsche's ideas of the 'will to power' and the *Übermensch*, the overman, who could justify humanity's existence and overcome and realize him- or herself, opposes any concept of realizing a pre-given essential self or inner child. For Heidegger, humans are beings whose being is in question, and there is no essence there. According to Heidegger, authenticity is an ongoing process and narrative of our own construction from an ineffable base upon which we actively attempt to realize our goals, including overarching long-term goals, whether we consciously adopt them or not. Laing characterized Heidegger's enigmatic conception of truth as 'that which is literally without secrecy' (Laing, 1969, p. 129).

Along the same lines, Jean-Paul Sartre suggested that the world can be divided into existence or being for itself on the one hand and essence or being in itself on the other. According to Sartre, only humans have the character of existence, and things have an essence (Sartre, 1948, p. 28).

Sartre mapped this central idea of a non-essential self as patterns of self-deception, based upon how we try to avoid the freedom to which we are all condemned. Authenticity means recognizing *not* having an essential pre-given false self, and this fact determines the patterns of inauthenticity. Sartre's clearest insights are about treating ourselves as agents, as choosing beings, not as things. According to Sartre, we often try to escape into seeing ourselves or others as things instead of as choosing beings with their own axes of orientation.

Sartre posited two kinds of being – being-in-itself and being-for-itself, being and nothingness – being as that which is, and nothingness as a gap in being, an indefinable free agent that can't get away from having to choose. Sartre sees self-deception *(mauvaise foi)* as a project that aims at escaping freedom. He proposes different patterns of self-deception in treating ourselves or others as objects or things. He instances a waiter who tries too hard in pretending to be a waiter, overacting the role of waiter almost as a caricature. Another example: the woman on a first date who pretends that her hand being grasped is not really her hand, something that is her, but instead a separate object out there in the world that things just happen to. She is trying to dissociate, to disown herself, to distance the action, to treat part of herself as a mechanistic object. Pretending not to be able to make choices is itself a choice, and dis-owning ourselves is inauthentic (Sartre, 1943[1984]).

Heidegger and Sartre don't prescribe how to behave so much as describe ways not to. Sartre's fictional trilogy of the 1940s, *The Roads to Freedom*, describes the paradoxes and complexities of different paths we pursue in evading our freedom and how authentic freedom can come only upon recognizing false ways of being, recognizing the paths not to go down (Sartre, 1961, 1963a, 1963b). That is an ethic of owning oneself and one's behavior and not dis-owning it.

As Heidegger suggests, we are the beings whose being is in question, and as Sartre puts it, we are condemned to freedom in that we are not free not to be free (Sartre, 1948, p. 34). Authenticity need not be a self-serving overvaluation of oneself. It can be transcending, reaching out beyond where one is to the world of others in terms of ful-filment of one's overarching projects in relationship between self and others. For both Heidegger and Sartre, authenticity lies in my owning up to my freedom and choices.

Laing sketches the ways we encumber ourselves or are framed by others into not seeing what is going on or not seeing the paths out from where we don't want to be.

Sartre thought choosing was unfathomable. But as choosing beings, we are sad-dled with having to choose and making our choices – for Sartre, we are our choices, we are our actions. For Sartre, we can change ourselves by changing our choices and actions while we are alive. At the same time as we irredeemably choose, we are also encumbered with commensurate and inescapable responsibility for our actions together with their consequences. We are what we do and cannot avoid bearing the consequences. In fact, I think that authenticity involves not only being responsible for your choices and actions but also not turning a blind eye to their probable con-sequences and taking them into account.

I have outlined Laing's indebtedness to the major existential thinkers whose thought formed the foundation of his approach to authenticity. Let us now look more directly at Laing's ideas. Because Laing does not often explicitly discuss authenticity as underlying his approach even though it is always implicit, it is not easy to directly examine it. Nonetheless, there are some clear indicators.

The Divided Self is based upon the assumption of authenticity. A science of persons for Laing explicitly recognized the difference between seeing somebody as a free human being and as a mechanism. The concepts of true and false self and false-self systems explain ways that people deceive themselves and others that they are not making choices. For Laing, mental illness is far more intelligible in terms of the meaning and choices patients make so that such choices can be deciphered, decoded, unmasked or unveiled. In *The Divided Self*, Laing draws on existentialist thinkers, particularly Sartre on self-deception, to explain the differences between explicit authentic choices and false and inauthentic choices, which can be revealed in terms of false-self confusions. According to Laing, the schizophrenic's vulner-able true self does not feel it is participating in the activities of the false-self sys-tems which mask it (Laing, 1965, p. 74).

For the Laing of *The Divided Self*, the psychotic is understood in terms of attempts to solve existential problems using the person's ineluctable freedom and subjectivity. In this Laing is a firm follower of Sartre. The hysteric's dissociations are, for Laing, best described as Sartre's concept of 'self-deception'. Laing sees much of schizophrenia as

> simply nonsense, red-herring speech, prolonged filibustering to throw danger-ous people off the scent, to create boredom and futility in others. The schizo-phrenic is often making a fool of himself and the doctor. He is playing at being mad to avoid at all costs the possibility of being held responsible for a single coherent idea, or intention.
>
> (Laing, 1965, p. 164)

This inauthentic behavior is seen to be more of a way out than usually thought. As Laing puts it, 'The false self is one way of not being'. He goes on to list several important existentialist studies 'relevant to understanding the false self as one way of living inauthentically' (1965, p. 94n).

To understand ourselves only from the vantage point of our consciousness of what is going on is normally to be mistaken. Authenticity is based on the nature of the unknown self, alignment with it and expression of it. How can we listen or pay attention to our-selves honestly and speak candidly? In a report of an undated lecture Laing delivered to the Department of Psychiatry at Trinity College Dublin, Laing cited Euripides from *The Phoenician Women*, 'A slave is a man who dares not speak his thoughts'.

Laing conveyed a romantic vision of schizophrenia in *The Politics of Experi-ence*. It even seemed at the time as though ordinary people were, as such, inauthen-tic and false, not just 'little boxes'. But neo-Marxist philosopher Herbert Marcuse suggested all of us in the first world were so alienated as to not recognize that we were alienated at all. In this situation, it seemed to Laing that somehow schizo-phrenics might be able to glimpse a way out into authenticity, albeit through a tiny pane of glass darkly. Although Laing contributed to the romanticization of mental illness as finding true selves and challenging false selves, he also mapped the nature of authenticity as agency and ways out of living alienated lives. On this basis, it is easy to see why for Laing mad people would stand out. However, the inner self is neither good nor bad, but ineffable, uncanny. This implies that the terms 'true' and 'false self' are confusing and misleading because neither one is exclusively true or false. For example, a false self may be a misnomer, as it is really a social self we need for getting along with others in daily living.

The paradoxes of freedom question the simple romantic notion of some kind of essential self. In my view, the Laing of *The Politics of Experience* traversed roman-tic Rousseauian territory by idealizing madness and seeing mad people as what his Kingsley Hall colleague Joe Berke labeled 'a sort of emotional proletariat' (Bev-eridge, 2011, p. 317). Laing gave credence to such romantic notions in *The Politics of Experience* where the split of Us and Them meant that We were good and They were bad and that schizophrenics were akin to Renaissance explorers (Laing, 1967). Mary Barnes's famous journey through madness was charted as a search for authenticity. I don't think anybody who knew Mary Barnes thought she succeeded that well.

Laing was allergic to anything fake or counterfeit. He reacted, even seriously over-reacted, to a sense of a lack of genuineness. But he really appreciated the genuine article and resonated with a genuine person, such as a schizophrenic patient with whom he was able to relate in a natural way. He liked plain speaking and wrote in words of one syllable.

Laing began and ended with individuality. He emphasized the values of authenticity, candidness, honesty, straightforwardness and being who you are without pretense. The idea of the asylum communities was that they were havens, crucibles of experience, where people could be themselves, often uncomfortably rubbing up against others, hopefully without harming them. It rested on the idea that people could be respected for being who they were. We need a community to be authentic.

On his tours of the United States in 1972, Laing recalls that he was often asked by students, 'How do we get in touch with our feelings?' (1976, p. 31). That degree of alienation from who we are, that we can be strangers to ourselves, was an alarm signal. This was a time when childbirth could be seen as simply a medical procedure under the gaze of a 'scientific look' and not as a meaningful life event (1976, p. 64).

He was very individualistic. Laing valued the individual highly as a unique being whom we couldn't presume to know at bottom. We are all different, and we can't read minds. Although we shouldn't presume to know what the other person is thinking, we can have a sense of it, how it seems to be.

Laing is, if you like, a methodological individualist. Along with other existentialists, he begins from the standpoint of the individual and their experience and then works outwards and upwards to more social and collective concepts. But, like Sartre, he never abandons the focus on the individual's experience and actions and the consequences of that stance within collective psychosocial systems. This is where authenticity is crucial to understanding the foundation of individual actions and interactions, labeling and the impacts of the social systems we inhabit. This was always a challenge. There is no pregiven fit, and Laing is far more Freud than Marx in his understanding of the inherent tensions in relationships and society that cannot be resolved. Laing begins with the intuitions of existentialists and respect for the individual's unique experience and agency. Sartre followed this path from individual through to social system, inquiring as to how it is possible to be authentic in systems in which we may not be aware of its rules, injunctions and structures. How can we situate choice within serial or nexal groups in which we live, such as the family?

However, for Laing, no individual is just an island and always exists within what Sartre would term a 'situation'. But their individuality is still there, even if constrained or alienated. The individual needs to be comprehended in context. Our consciousness is always consciousness of something. That context is the internal context of different and mostly unconscious aspects of self. But that context needs to be comprehended within the relationship of self and other. Again, self and other are situated within a family or group context, and the family exists within the system of society and that within the total social world system. That world, again, exists within a spiritual or cosmological context. Much of Laing's work lies avowedly in the zone of communications theory and research exploring the possibility of mapping the patterns of relationships in the human world and investigating how we might be able to see the ground clearly enough to individually flourish. This approach involves understanding and revealing from the position of the individual not only the rules of the game but the meta-rules, meta-meta-rules and so on.

If we don't know who we are, at least we might know some of the things we aren't. We will always act with limited knowledge, given factors such as the unconscious and impacts that we are not aware of. We can do the best we can, honestly, straightforwardly, owning up to the responsibility for our actions.

I will now outline Laing's only explicit and albeit brief discussion about his approach to authenticity.

In *Self and Others* Laing gets to the heart of what inauthentic or alienated action is. It is about putting oneself into a false or untenable position or being put into such positions. Laing equates inauthenticity with what he calls being in a false existential position. He cites colloquialisms and everyday speech that demonstrate our experience of place and position in our world. A person can put himself or herself 'into' their acts or may not be 'in' them. Or a person may 'lose' or 'forget himself' or be 'full of himself' or 'beside himself', all attributions about the person's relation to their own actions. In all of them the issue is

> the extent to which the act is seen or felt to *potentiate* the being or existence of the doer, or the extent to which the action . . . makes patent the latent self of the doer.
>
> (Laing, 1969, p. 126)

Laing suggests that we feel we are going forward when we put ourselves into our actions, 'when we disclose or make patent our true self'. Or we may be liable to feel that we are 'going back', 'going round in circles', or 'getting nowhere'. Thus, Laing submits,

> In 'putting myself into' what I do, I lose myself, and in so doing I seem to become myself. The act I do is felt to be me, and I become 'me' in and through such action. Also, there is a sense in which a person 'keeps himself alive' by his acts; each act can be a new beginning, a new birth, a recreation of oneself.
>
> (Laing, 1969, p. 126)

In a rare direct comment on authenticity, Laing goes on to explain,

> To be 'authentic' is to be true to oneself, to be what one is, to be 'genuine'. To be 'inauthentic' is to not be oneself, to be false to oneself: to be not as one appears to be, to be counterfeit. We tend to link the categories of truth and reality by saying that a genuine act is real, but that a person who habitually uses action as a masquerade is not real.
>
> (1969, p. 127)

Laing sees the self-disclosure of authenticity as being what Nietzsche meant by the 'will to power'. Laing explains,

> It is the 'weak' man who, in lieu of potentiating himself genuinely, counter-feits his impotence by dominating and controlling others, by idealizing physical strength or sexual potency.

For Laing, I may feel fulfilled by an 'act that is genuine, revealing, and potenti-ating' in 'an act that is me: in this action I am myself. I put myself "in" it. In so far as I put myself "into" what I do, I become myself through this doing'. Conversely, I feel empty when it is not my doing (Laing, 1969, p. 127).

Citing Heidegger, Laing contrasts two notions of truth. First, there is the natural scientific concept that consists of the correspondence of what goes on in the mind and what happens in the world. The second notion of truth derives from the pre-Socratic concept of *Alethia*, which is that which is without secrecy, what discloses itself without a veil (Laing, 1969, p. 129).

What if the inauthentic person, the person in a false position, isn't aware of being 'in' such a position? The person can only experience his or her position as false to the extent that he or she is not totally estranged from their 'own' experience and actions.

Laing vividly describes the consequences of this false position of inauthenticity:

> Perhaps without his realizing it his 'life' comes to a stop. With no real future of his own, he may be in that supreme despair which is, as Kierkegaard says, not to know he is in despair. He is in despair because he has lost 'his own' future, and so can have no genuine hope or trust in any future. The person in a false position has lost a starting-point of his own from which to throw or thrust himself, that is, to project himself, forward. He has lost the place. He does not know where he is or where he is going. He cannot get anywhere however hard he tries. In despair, just as one place is the same as another, so one time is the same as another. The future is the resultant of the present, the present is the resultant of the past, and past is unalterable.
>
> (Laing, 1969, p. 131)

This is not a good way to be. Although authenticity can be an uncomfortable way to be, it can have its rewards in terms of being alive, real, genuine, a sense of being one's own unique self and ownership of actions and better relationships.

However, authenticity comes at a cost. It goes with being confronted and living with the human condition, the world which Freud outlined in *Civilization and Its Discontents*: the inevitable pain and suffering of life, the realities of our vulnerabil-ity to our own bodies, other people, the perils of nature and mortality.

And there are the perils of authenticity. What is the cost of being authentic, of authenticity? It can make us uncomfortable and incapable of being honest with a real fear of other people, especially in a politically correct or more directly oppressive society. There is no pat answer here – it's a balance. How much authenticity can we get away with? Can it be authentic then to go along to get along? Such questions go to the heart of Laing's interrogatory perspective.

References

Beveridge, A. (2011). *Portrait of the psychiatrist as a young man: The early writing and work of R. D. Laing, 1927–1960*. Oxford: Oxford University Press.

Charlesworth, M. (1973). *The existentialists and Jean-Paul Sartre*. St Lucia: University of Queensland Press.

Heidegger, M. (1927[1962]). *Being and time* (J. Macquarrie and E. Robinson, Trans.). Oxford: Basil Blackwell.

Laing, R. D. (1965). *The divided self: An existential study in sanity and madness*. Harmondsworth: Penguin Books (Original edition 1960).

Laing, R. D. (1967). *The politics of experience and the bird of paradise*. Harmondsworth: Penguin Books.

Laing, R. D. (1969). *Self and others*. Harmondsworth: Penguin Books.

Laing, R. D. (1976). *The facts of life: An essay in feelings, facts, and fantasy*. New York: Pantheon.

Mill, J. S. (1863). *Utilitarianism*. www.utilitarianism.com/mill2.htm

Sartre, J.-P. (1943[1984]). *Being and nothingness* (Hazel E. Barnes, Trans.). New York: Washington Square Press.

Sartre, J.-P. (1948). *Existentialism and humanism*. London: Methuen.

Sartre, J.-P. (1961). *The age of reason*. Harmondsworth: Penguin Books.

Sartre, J.-P. (1963a). *The reprieve*. Harmondsworth: Penguin Books.

Sartre, J.-P. (1963b). *Iron in the soul*. Harmondsworth: Penguin Books.

Chapter 14

The Dark Side of Authenticity

Laing as Provocateur

M. Guy Thompson, PhD

In this essay I want to focus on the undeniably controversial aspects of Laing's efforts to adopt as authentic a manner as he could in both his clinical and his extra-clinical, including collegial, relationships, even his friendships. What I am about to share with you is not based on Laing's published work, where he said little about his conception of authenticity as such. Instead, I will base my remarks on Laing's relationship with authenticity from my personal relationship with him over the course of some seventeen years, from the time I met him in 1972 until his death in 1989. I first came to really know Laing in 1973 when I moved to London to study with him at his school, the Philadelphia Association, over a period of seven years. After I returned to California in 1980, I enjoyed occasional visits from Laing at my home in Berkeley until his untimely death in 1989. So I knew Laing in a variety of contexts: as my boss when I was the administrator of his organization and as my teacher, supervisor, friend, house guest, and confidante. Over the course of these sixteen-plus years I observed Laing in all kinds of circumstances, both professional and personal. During that time we happened to discuss his views about authenticity on numerous occasions, as well as countless other topics, many of which he did not disclose in his many publications. So what I share with you now is for the most part distilled from these reminiscences.

I should warn you that what I am about to share with you will be of a both positive and negative nature, because Laing was both a sensitive and loving human being, on the one hand, but a man who could also be brutal and confrontational, if not exactly wicked. Laing made no bones about this. One of the things I admired most about him was that Laing never put himself out as a saint, or even a role model. He readily acknowledged that he was a sinner. One of the things I admired about him most was his honesty, which was at the very heart of his authenticity. His struggle to determine the nature of authenticity, to define precisely what he believed it entails, and to measure up to that standard himself brought out the best and the worst in him, as everyone who knew Laing personally discovered, sometimes to shocking effect.

Laing's conception of authenticity relied predominantly on the thinking of Friedrich Nietzsche, Martin Heidegger, and especially Jean-Paul Sartre. These are the three European philosophers to whom we are all indebted for the most radical – and,

DOI: 10.4324/9781003564294-19

for many, disturbing – conceptions of authenticity in a sea of more recent and competing versions of it that bear little resemblance to how Laing himself conceived it. Kierkegaard was also a seminal influence, whom I will turn to later. In order to understand Laing's unorthodox take on what it means to be authentic and the extremes of behavior that Laing believed epitomizes this concept, it would help to familiarize ourselves with Nietzsche's, Heidegger's, and Sartre's respective views on this philosophical principle.

The popular notion of authenticity that has swept contemporary America in recent years tends to characterize it as more or less whatever one happens to *feel*, as opposed to what is occurring in one's head. This view goes all the way back to Rousseau in the Enlightenment era, where he challenged the views of other Enlightenment thinkers, who emphasized the life of the mind. We often think of the Enlightenment period, which began in the eighteenth century, as the birthplace of modern science. Rousseau also valued science greatly, but he was of the opinion that his colleagues privileged science too much at the expense of *feeling states* that were of crucial importance to artists, musicians, novelists, and the like. Rousseau proposed that all human beings possess an inner self that is hidden from others and comprises feelings that say more about who that person is than who they often "think," or believe, they are. This suggests that the more in touch you are with your feelings, the more in touch with your inner self you are, which Rousseau believed is the most authentic or genuine aspect of our nature. Another implication of this argument is that the more authentic a person is, the more ethical that person will be in relation to others and to society in general. In other words, the authentic person, according to the contemporary perspective, is a kinder, gentler person than the person who is inauthentic. The inauthentic person may pretend to be loving and kind and fool many people into believing this about them, but what that person is hiding from others is dark and implicitly objectionable. Carl Rogers is the contemporary champion of this version of authenticity.

Neither Nietzsche, nor Heidegger, nor Sartre would have agreed with this perspective. There are many reasons for this. First, they did not believe in the notion of a substantial self, hidden or otherwise, so there is no "inner core" of feelings that one can get in or out of touch with. Moreover, there is no direct or necessary relationship between authenticity and morality, if by morality we believe in a universal code of conduct that structures desirable behavior. In the view of Sartre, Nietzsche, or Heidegger, the authentic person may well be an anarchist or a rebel whose vision of society is anathema to prevailing opinion. In fact, behaving authentically may result in becoming extremely unpopular, as all three of these existentialists have demonstrated in their personal conduct.

Nietzsche, for example, insisted that the authentic individual is a person who is not afraid of her desires and has the courage to live her life with passion, whatever the consequences may be. Such a person was embodied in Nietzsche's concept of the *Übermensch*, usually translated into English as overman or superman. This person couldn't care less about public opinion and would be relatively fearless in devising the trajectory that his life should follow, as well as the code he will live by. Though Nietzsche rejected the conventional view of morality – that we should conduct ourselves by a set of rules dictated by God, public opinion, or political legislation – he nevertheless embraced certain values that the *Übermensch* should, in fact, live by. He believed, for example, that *courage* and *honesty* are by far the most important virtues that the authentic person should cultivate. Nietzsche saw the *Übermensch* as a heroic figure, because it takes a lot of courage to go against the herd and follow the beat of your own drum, which is exactly how Nietzsche conducted his relatively short life.

It is telling that Laing's most famous and polemical book, *The Politics of Experience* (1967), where he railed against modern society as a toxic wasteland, is an *homage* to Nietzsche's *Thus Spoke Zarathustra*, as well as Freud's *Civilization and Its Discontents*, two of Laing's favorite books. Courage is a theme to which Laing referred countless times, noting that etymologically, its root goes back to the Latin *cor*, meaning "heart." This suggests that the literal meaning of courage is not bravery, but "openheartedness," which for Nietzsche entails passion. Laing would agree that it takes courage be authentic, because it involves opening one's heart to another person, perhaps the riskiest endeavor any human being can undertake. Consistent with this line of thinking, Laing interpreted Kierkegaard's (1956) concept of authenticity as an edition of *agapé*, the Greek word for selfless or spiritual love (see Chapter 10).

Heidegger's conception of authenticity shares similarities with Nietzsche's, but with the exception that Heidegger believed all human beings are inherently *inauthentic* most of the time, because this is the human condition from which we cannot escape. We are, however, capable of acting authentically when circumstances challenge us to do so for the sake of our integrity. The rest of the time we get caught up in the pursuit of our daily business, going along with the flow of life in more or less inauthentic fashion in the way, for example, that we court popular favor, compete for promotions, seek to cultivate our reputations, and shamelessly engage in lying when being truthful may prove too embarrassing. In other words, we get caught up "in the crowd" of our own making, whatever crowd or circle we adopt as our own, and this crowd becomes the arena of our inauthenticity as well as our self-identity. But it is also a source of our estrangement from *ourselves*, and when our inauthenticity is excessive, it elicits a sense of guilt about pretending to be someone that we are not.

From Heidegger one gets the sense that we are imperfect, fallen creatures, suffering from a profound homelessness that we can never entirely overcome. This is because remaining faithful to your principles and doing what you believe is right will sometimes cost you job opportunities, financial success, and even friends who expect you to abandon your principles and devote yourself to their agenda. Can a person who embraces authenticity, for example, be intimate with someone who embraces inauthenticity as a matter of course? This question had a profound impact on Laing's thoughts about love. It may also account for why he had few friends. Yet Laing could be uncommonly forgiving of his own, as well as others,' failings. One of the most novel aspects of Laing's conception of authenticity was his belief that the wherewithal to be honest about your inauthentic transgressions was almost as "authentic" as behaving authentically!

Yet of all the existential philosophers, Laing probably resonated most closely with Sartre. They were closer in age, and Sartre admired Laing's views on psychiatry and his efforts to reform it. Sartre probably took the concept of authenticity further than any other philosopher, even rejecting the marital contract and bourgeois society's mores, especially its flagrant materialism. Sartre was uncompromising in his own definition of what authenticity entails and resonated with Heidegger's argument that all of us are condemned to live our lives in *bad faith*, Sartre's term for inauthenticity. Sartre explained that the reason for this is because each of us is born free and condemned to remain so, which means each of us is responsible for who we are and how we get on in the world. Like Nietzsche, Sartre believed we must *live* our desire and that we do so passionately. Sartre was the most famous of the existentialist thinkers and a prolific novelist and playwright who was awarded the Nobel Prize for Literature. Laing, at that time the world's best-selling psychiatrist, no doubt resonated with this aspect of Sartre's notoriety. That Laing and Sartre never became friends, however, was a bitter disappointment to him.

So what were the basic elements of authenticity in Laing's thinking? Laing couldn't stand people who he thought were "fake," who put on airs and pretended to be who they were not, and were too shy to speak up for fear of making a fool of themselves, or when they tried to impress you. On the other hand he loved it when you just came out and tried, however pathetically, to be yourself. This wasn't an easy thing to do in Laing's presence, because Laing was never really comfortable with people, and his discomfort was palpable. A lot of Laing's preoccupation with the nature of the true and false self in *The Divided Self* (1960) speaks to his preoccupation with the inherent *falsity* that people erect around themselves in order to fit in with society. In effect, they pretend to be someone they aren't and then get confused as to who they really are. Both Winnicott and Sartre were influences in Laing's adoption of this language. Though Laing used this terminology in his early work, he discarded it as his thinking evolved, though he never wavered from his distaste for what he termed "putting on airs." Laing could be confrontational and, to some, even cruel in the way he could get in your face and call you out on something, a tactic he borrowed from Esalen encounter groups that he participated in on his many visits there in the 1960a, 1970s, and 1980s.

Yet Laing could just as easily be uncommonly gentle, kind, and compassionate. It all depended on what you drew out of him in the moment. Laing was also spiritual in his way. The most important litmus for his personal stamp on authenticity derived from the Golden Rule: Do unto others as you would have them do to you. I can't think of another expression that I heard Laing utter more than this one in terms of basic human decency, as a rough and ready guide to authentic relating. In the seminars I helped organize he would sometimes read from the Lord's Prayer, influenced by a book of Aldous Huxley's, where he goes through each line of the prayer, giving it a contemporary interpretation. He was particularly taken with the part of the prayer that speaks of *trespassing* against one's neighbors and the need to forgive those who trespass against oneself as well as one's own trespasses against them, in turn. Laing seemed especially sensitive to crossing that line, when therapists, for example, may unwittingly intrude into that space of vulnerability that is not necessarily therapeutic, but injurious. This seems to be the one irreducible element of Laing's critique of psychiatry, as well as other therapeutic practices. In his critique of contemporary mental health mores, Laing didn't seem to care how many psychiatrists and psychoanalysts he offended, and he paid a price for speaking out against the kinds of manipulative clinical interventions that even today we take for granted. The psychiatric establishment still hasn't forgiven him for it. I consider this pretty heroic stuff, but it only paints part of the picture, and to be honest, the more interesting part of the picture is a bit disturbing.

What are we to make of a man who at the time of his death had managed to alienate most of his closest friends and colleagues as a consequence of his unforgivably hostile and grievous behavior, who delighted in bullying those closest to him as a form of sport, whose drinking and drug use drove him to behaving so irresponsibly over the last decade of his life that it was obvious to those closest to him that he was gradually destroying a reputation that had taken him only a few years in the 1960s to cultivate? For those of us who knew Laing and loved him, witnessing this process was painful, and nearly every one of us fell victim at one time or other to this behavior, depending on his state of inebriation.

Despite Laing's efforts to equate authenticity with not trespassing on others, Laing sometimes engaged in behavior that to some crossed that very line he accused the psychiatric establishment of. How can we reconcile Laing's unseemly behavior with the very conception of authenticity that he tried to justify it with? In other words, was Laing's penchant for bullying a form of unmitigated rudeness masquerading as being honest or a manifestation of genuine authentic self-expression, true to his personal values, but not easy to understand or appreciate at the moment?

As I was writing this essay I was glancing through some of the contributions to Bob Mullan's collection of papers about Laing that was published shortly after his death in the early 1990s, one of which I contributed. This collection consisted of articles and testimonials by some of Laing's friends and cohorts, all of whom knew him in varying degrees of intimacy. Many of the contributions were reverential, but what struck me most going through them was the pain expressed even by some who were closest to him. Saddest was no doubt the contribution from John Duffy, Laing's oldest and dearest friend from childhood. John Duffy described Laing as a kind and loving young man, a really outstanding individual who was different from the rest, profoundly caring and gentle. In his contribution Duffy said that Laing changed over time and became increasingly self-absorbed and sometimes brutal. Some of this he attributed to his first and extremely unhappy marriage to Anne. But later when Laing married Jutta and became famous, despite Duffy's observation that this marriage was happier than the first, his brutal behavior escalated and encroached into their friendship. He said that Laing's drinking escalated and he became increasingly aggressive and belligerent over time. Duffy recounts an incident at a local bar in Scotland when Laing threw a glass of whisky at a barmaid for no apparent reason. What finally got to Duffy, however, was Laing's increasing self-absorption. Their conversations were always about *his* pain, with less and less time apportioned for concern about Duffy's, until he finally concluded that Laing simply didn't care about his friend any more. Eventually he had enough and ended their friendship, much to Laing's consternation.

Everyone who knew Laing had experienced what Duffy was talking about first-hand: the drinking, the anger, the bullying and aggression, crossing the line – in a word, *trespassing*. Yet Laing would often argue that it wasn't simply a case of being drunk or out of control, that there was method to his madness, in the tradition of William Blake whose famous adage *The road of excess leads to the palace of wisdom*. Such accounts could be confusing because Laing could just as readily apologize for such behavior as if to say he didn't mean it, while on other occasions he would insist, in a paranoid kind of way, that he was provoked or was teaching someone a lesson.

An example of this latter explanation was recounted by Maureen O'Hara, an ex-patriot British woman who had been living in Southern California for some years working with Carl Rogers as a personal assistant. In 1978 O'Hara contacted Laing's organization proposing a one-day public event featuring Laing and Rogers, who was planning to visit London. As the organization's administrator, I was assigned to work with O'Hara and organize the event which eventually took place at the London Hilton. A coterie of followers who accompanied Rogers and a group of people who Laing selected from his cohorts were to participate in an all-day workshop, titled **An Encounter with Carl Rogers and R. D. Laing**. The event itself was uneventful, but the evening before was a night the participants will never forget. Laing and Rogers had never met, so he invited Rogers's group to his home the evening before the workshop to get acquainted and to plan their presentation. But from the moment they arrived at Laing's doorstep, in O'Hara's words, an air of discomfort pervaded the room. Rogers's group introduced themselves while Laing, Hugh Crawford, and others sat by in stony silence saying nothing until Rogers's group had finished. This was followed by more silence. Finally, as the silence became unbearable, Laing announced to Rogers: "If you and I are to have any kind of meaningful dialogue, you are going to have to cut out the California 'nice-guy' act and get to something approaching an authentic encounter."

At this point a testy exchange of views concerning the human condition was shared, Rogers with his everyone-has-love-at-their-core perspective, while Laing's group proceeded to expound the opposite view, that it is probably the "nice" people in the world who are most responsible for the mess the world is in. After this exchange began to fall apart, the two groups were more polarized than ever and began insulting each other. Laing decided it was time to break for dinner. At a restaurant near his home, Laing isolated himself from the others and proceeded to drink whisky, much to Rogers's and his group's discomfort. Then a handful of strangers entered the restaurant and Laing suddenly called out to them: "See that bald-headed man over there" – pointing to Rogers – "well, he's not really a man, he's a *perrrson!*" – alluding to Rogers's most famous book, *On Becoming a*

Person, in an unmistakably sarcastic fashion with his famous Scottish burr. As the room fell into stunned silence, Laing ambled over to where O'Hara was sitting and proceeded to pour some whisky into her empty water glass. He asked if she liked it and she said she did, thinking this was a gesture of friendly camaraderie designed to defuse the tension. At this point Laing spat in her drink and then asked, "Well, how do you like it now?" O'Hara tossed the drink in his face and the situation devolved into pandemonium. Everyone fled the restaurant, and once outside the two groups were on the verge of a fist fight. Laing announced that the Rogers group was not welcome to return to his home. At this point Rogers's group announced they were withdrawing from the event, scheduled for the very next morning.

Though the groups eventually patched things up and went on with the program, a considerable amount of damage had been done. Later, Laing held to his conviction that making Rogers and his group feel intensely uncomfortable by insulting and provoking them was his way of breaking them out of their shell and behaving more authentically which, after all, was the topic of their presentation. He was goading them into becoming "real" in a way that they were not being with him and his group, because they were busy being so "nice," but, in Laing's view, artificial. Rogers had cut his teeth on his own conception of authenticity, and Laing thought he needed a lesson or two. So he decided to get the group rattled and angry with him in order to show them what they were made of, the rot, as it were, beneath the sweet facade, which came out when they finally exploded. Laing insisted that anything goes when it comes to stripping away this kind of artificial niceness, whenever and wherever one meets it, no matter how much trespassing is needed. I don't believe in Laing's right mind that he entirely believed this, but that he fell prey to such behavior on certain occasions when he was in a state of despair. To his credit, he never behaved that way with his patients, only his friends and colleagues!

Yet not everything is as it seems. To give Laing his due, O'Hara's conclusion to this story is perhaps most surprising. Despite the disappointment and incomprehension that Rogers felt toward Laing, for O'Hara, it was a life-changing experience. After returning to Laing's home to patch things up, O'Hara suffered a breakdown from the stress and strain of the evening, which culminated in a profound therapeutic experience that was life-changing. After she returned to the United States she began to see Rogers in a new light. Previously she had idolized him and believed strongly in his message. In fact, he had used her as his mistress while traveling away from his wife, and she decided she was fed up with it. After the experience at Laing's home she said that she realized that she no longer needed Rogers as a crutch and that she was now able to stand on her own feet. She had suffered a crisis but was able to take a step forward in her self-development, feeling wiser and self-confident for the first time. All apparently due to the way Laing had challenged them that evening. Was Laing's "authentic" behavior an agent of therapeutic change or merely a coincidence?

Laing was a mass of contradictions. He was a solitary figure with a profoundly spiritual center that fueled his quest for authentic relating with both himself and with others, especially with people in his care. Yet he pursued fame and notoriety with such zeal that you would have thought his life depended on the adulation of strangers. Laing once confided to my six-year old son on a visit to Berkeley that from the time he was a child he had a singular, burning ambition: *To grow up to be healthy, wealthy, and wise . . . AND rich and famous!* Fame emerged as the driving force in his life, a quest that virtually tore him apart because it couldn't have been more antithetical to a person who was committed to a path of wisdom and authentic relating. Laing hated being famous but couldn't live without it. He often recounted his tortuous, loveless relationship with his mother who was obsessed with him but also bent on destroying him. I concluded that his quest for fame was a desperate attempt to win love from any quarter but without having to reciprocate. This is perhaps what drives all famous people to be special, to get the love that was hard to come by in their families.

Laing despised the people who came to his lectures and bought his books because he believed – quite rightly, I think – that most of them hadn't a clue what his message was about and didn't care. They were drawn to him *because* he was famous, not *why* he was famous. Yet from the early 1970s Laing's ability to write in the way he had in the 1960's collapsed as his books became increasingly self-referential and an embarrassment to those of us who worked with him and, frankly, expected more. This was the period of time during which I came to know Laing, the 1970s, the beginning of his decline. By 1980, the year I left London to return to California, it was evident that he was never going to write that last "great book" that everyone kept waiting for, to redeem both himself and his complicated legacy.

It is perhaps ironic that Laing's last book, which he was unable to finish, was devoted to love, a topic that was central to his conception of authenticity, yet a topic that I often suspected tormented him. Heidegger allowed that none of us are perfect and that we cannot be authentic all or even much of the time, that simply being honest about our limitations is often the most honorable option at our disposal.[1] Yet Laing argued that while love is central to authentic relating to others and that *caritas*, or charity, is the most profound kind of love – because it is the most self-effacing – he also argued that hatred is perfectly consistent with loving. Even acts of cruelty may be consistent with an authentic way of relating to a person, depending on the context.

In his biography of Laing, John Clay notes that Laing used to have a painting of Breughel's *Fall of Icarus* hanging on the wall of his consulting room on Wimpole Street in the early days of his psychoanalytic practice. Anthony Clare interprets Laing's choice of this famous Greek myth as especially apt in that Laing also flew too close to the sun as a consequence of his elevation to the status of a guru. Laing desperately needed people to love him, and those of us who knew him knew of the loneliness he endured as a child, the depression he struggled with throughout his life, and his disappointment with his own analysis at finding relief from the torment he suffered on a day-to-day basis. Drugs and alcohol were a constant, but the real drug that he couldn't do without was the worship of other people. This was the narcissistic component of Laing's personality. The decline of his status in the 1980s as it intersected with the end of his marriage to Jutta resulted in a crisis that led to his leaving the UK and becoming an intellectual nomad without a home. He went through a period of acting out that severed his relationship with his organization and cost him his medical license, which he surrendered when he chose not to submit to an inquiry that was triggered by a complaint against him. He spent the last six years of his life on the road without a home base, at the mercy of the public he so despised to financially support him with the revenue from lectures he gave all over the globe, often in an inebriated condition. As he told me on one of his visits to California during this period, "These people are not paying for a coherent lecture, something they can ponder and think about. They're paying for nothing more than to see *R. D. Laing* – so by God, that's what they're going to get . . . warts and all!"

I think that even in these acts of rebelliousness Laing was trying his best to salvage what was left of his capacity to remain authentic in the face of having sold out to a forum that he had nothing but contempt for. Maybe there was a grain of truth to this? He had opportunities for employment during this time that he was exploring in the form of university posts, one of which was the Hoover Institute at Stanford University. Something was arranged through Rollo May and Carl Rogers, who had forgiven him for the London experience and considered him a friend. All Laing had to do was to show up, be sober . . . and be nice. Something, we know, that did not come naturally. When the time came, he just couldn't do it. He showed up drunk and blew the interview with his belligerence. So that was that. He didn't get the job. I actually admired this about Laing, his inability to grovel, to act the part. So long as this hurts no one but himself I still see something heroic in his inability to pander to the crowd. I think I love Laing for this and will always admire him for it. When it comes to crossing the line, trespassing on others in the guise of teaching them something about how to behave more authentically, I'm not so sure. I sometimes suspect that Laing engaged in acts of aggression that are difficult to reconcile with his views about *caritas*, peace on earth, and the like. But I also believe that Laing was a genius and perhaps his manner of teaching was simply over our heads?

Laing's last years were not easy. His popularity ebbed, and people actually thought he was dead. I suppose in some ways he was. But his decline was also on a deeper, spiritual level. Laing's father suffered from dementia and died in mental hospital. Laing suffered most of his adult life from the fear that he was prone to the same Scottish involutional melancholia that had afflicted his father and grandfather before him. He often wondered if he, too, would one day go stark-raving mad. Some thought he was already dying from an undiagnosed malady on that fateful day in St. Tropez when his life came to a sudden end on a tennis court under a searing afternoon sun, struck down by a heart attack. Yet however complicated and contradictory Laing's legacy remains, I owe him a debt I will never be able to repay. And the world, despite its having moved away from environmental explanations for the causes of psychotic disturbance, owes him a debt of gratitude for bringing the treatment of the mentally disturbed from the back wards of mental hospitals onto the front covers of newspapers and magazines where they have remained ever since. Despite his faults and, at times, questionable behavior, he was also, as his old friend Rollo May once remarked, "On the side of the angels."

Note

1 The English words "honest" and "honorable" have the same root, the Latin *honestus*, which is a fascinating word. Today, we typically use the word honest to connote a person who does not tell a lie, as in, "Are you being honest with me?" But the root word here is *honorable*. To be honest is merely a shorthand to an honorable person; a person of good moral character; who is virtuous, sincere, candid; a person who will not steal, or lie, or cheat, or betray you. In a word, a person you can count on to do the right thing. This is what the Yiddish word *mensch*, connotes. We don't really have a term in English that covers all these attributes in a person. The way we typically employ the word honest hardly covers it. And the word honorable sounds rather vague, doesn't it? However, the word *authentic* comes pretty close to nailing it.

References

Kierkegaard, S. (1956). *Purity of heart is to will one thing* (Douglas V. Steere, Trans.). New York: Harper and Row.

Laing, R. D. (1960). *The divided self*. London: Tavistock Books.

Laing, R. D. (1967). *The politics of experience*. New York: Pantheon Books.

Nietzsche, F. (1966). *Thus spoke Zarathustra: A book for all and none* (Walter Kaufman, Trans.). New York: The Viking Press.

Chapter 15

Authentic Community

Fritjof Capra, PhD

Community was a major theme in R. D. Laing's thinking and in his work, exemplified by the unique therapeutic communities he created in the 1960s and 1970s. In this essay, I want to discuss community from a systemic perspective; more specifically, from the perspective of what I call the systems view of life. This is a new understanding of life that has emerged in science during the last thirty years.

The Systems View of Life

At the forefront of contemporary science, the universe is no longer seen as a machine composed of elementary building blocks. We have discovered that the material world, ultimately, is a network of inseparable patterns of relationships; that the planet as a whole is a living, self-regulating system. The view of the human body as a machine and of the mind as a separate entity is being replaced by one that sees not only the brain but also the immune system, the bodily tissues, and even each cell as a living, cognitive system. Evolution is no longer seen as a competitive struggle for existence, but rather as a cooperative dance in which creativity and the constant emergence of novelty are the driving forces. And with the new emphasis on complexity, networks, and patterns of organization, a new science of qualities is slowly emerging.

During the last thirty years, I developed a synthesis of this new understanding of life; a conceptual framework that integrates four dimensions of life: the biological, the cognitive, the social, and the ecological dimension. I presented summaries of this framework as it evolved in several books. My final synthesis is published in a textbook titled *The Systems View of Life* coauthored with Pier Luigi Luisi, professor of biochemistry in Rome (Capra and Luisi, 2014).

I call my synthesis "the systems view of life" because it involves a new kind of thinking – thinking in terms of relationships, patterns, and context. In science, this way of thinking is known as "systemic thinking," or "systems thinking."

Living Networks

One of the most important insights of the systemic understanding of life is the recognition that networks are the basic pattern of organization of all living systems.

DOI: 10.4324/9781003564294-20

Ecosystems are understood in terms of food webs (i.e., networks of organisms); organism are networks of cells, organs, and organ systems; and cells are networks of molecules. The network is a pattern that is common to all life. Wherever we see life, we see networks. Indeed, at the very heart of the change of paradigms from the mechanistic to the systemic view of life, we find a fundamental change of metaphors: from seeing the world as a machine to understanding it as a network.

Now, a network, as everybody knows, is a certain pattern of links, of relationships. Therefore, to understand networks, we need to be able to think in terms of relationships and patterns. This is what systems thinking is all about.

Closer examination of these living networks has shown that their key characteristic is that they are *self-generating*. In a cell, for example, all the biological structures – the proteins, enzymes, the DNA, the cell membrane, etc. – are continually produced, repaired, and regenerated by the cellular network. Similarly, at the level of a multicellular organism, the bodily cells are continually regenerated and recycled by the organism's metabolic network. Living networks continually regenerate themselves by transforming or replacing their components. In this way they undergo continual structural changes while preserving their web-like patterns of organization. This coexistence of stability and change is indeed one of the key characteristics of life.

Life in the social realm can also be understood in terms of networks, but here we are not dealing with chemical reactions; we are dealing with communications. Social networks are networks of communications. Like biological networks, they are self-generating, but what they generate is mostly nonmaterial. Each communication creates thoughts and meaning, which give rise to further communications, and thus the entire network generates itself.

Culture and Community

As communications continue in a social network, they form multiple feedback loops which eventually produce a shared system of beliefs and values, known as culture, which is continually sustained by further communications. Through this culture individuals acquire identities as members of the social network, and in this way the network generates its own boundary. It is not a physical boundary, but a boundary of expectations, of confidentiality and loyalty, which is continually maintained and renegotiated by the network.

We can also say that as communications continue in a social network, they will generate a community. In the past, I used the terms "social network" and "community" interchangeably. But more recently I have come to realize that not every social network is a community. A community arises when there is a shared set of beliefs and values, a shared culture.

Community and Sustainability

There are several reasons for the importance of community in our time. One of our great challenges is to create and nurture sustainable communities, designed in such a way that their ways of life – businesses, economies, physical structures, and technologies – do not interfere with nature's inherent ability to sustain life. Over the last few years, I have become more and more convinced that the focus on community itself will be critical in this endeavor.

To design sustainable human communities, we first need to understand how nature sustains life. Over billions of years, the Earth's ecosystems have evolved certain patterns of organization to sustain the web of life. Examples of these patterns of organization are as follows: one species' waste is another species' food; matter cycles continually through the web of life; the energy driving the ecological cycles flows from the sun; diversity assures resilience. Most importantly, perhaps, we need to understand that life, from its beginning more than three billion years ago, did not take over the planet by combat, but by networking. These basic patterns of organization, or principles of ecology, can also be understood as principles of community.

Sustainability, then, is not an individual property, but a property of an entire web of relationships. It always involves a whole community. This is the profound lesson we need to learn from nature. The way to sustain life is to build and nurture communities. A sustainable human community interacts with other communities – human and nonhuman – in ways that enable them to live and develop according to their nature.

Today, the greatest obstacle to moving toward sustainability is the persistent illusion, maintained by most economists and politicians, that unlimited growth is possible on a finite planet. Economic and corporate growth are pursued relentlessly by promoting excessive material consumption. A continual barrage of advertising tells us that buying more goods will make us happier. The most powerful antidote against this corporate onslaught is to find happiness not in material consumption, but in human relationships – in other words, in community.

Communities of Practice

Building communities is important not only in our society at large but also within business organizations. The systems view of life tells us that living social systems are self-generating networks of communications. This means that a human organization will be a living system only if it is organized as a network or contains smaller networks within its boundaries. Indeed, organizational theorists have come to realize that informal social networks exist within every organization. They arise from various alliances and friendships, informal channels of communication, and other webs of relationships that continually grow, change, and adapt to new situations. Organizational theorists have called these informal networks "communities of practice."

Within every organization, there is a cluster of interconnected communities of practice. The more people are engaged in these informal networks and the more developed and sophisticated the networks are, the better the organization will be able to learn, respond creatively to unexpected new circumstances, change, and evolve. In other words, the organization's aliveness resides in its communities of practice. This is why the understanding of community is critical in the management of human organizations.

Community and Ethics

Now let us return to the challenge of ecological sustainability. I have mentioned the obsession with unlimited growth and material consumption as one of the main obstacles. Another big obstacle is the lack of a moral compass in our corporate and political world. Today, politics is dominated by economics – by corporate economics, to be precise. The so-called "global market," strictly speaking, is not a market at all, but a network of machines, of computers, programmed according to a single value – money-making for the sake of making money – to the exclusion of all other values. In other words, the global economy has been designed in such a way that all ethical dimensions are excluded. To build a sustainable future, it will be important to reintroduce ethics into economics and politics.

Ethics is usually associated with philosophy or religion, but it can also be considered from a scientific perspective. Throughout the long history of evolution, nature has sustained life by creating and nurturing communities, as I have mentioned. As soon as the first cells appeared on Earth, they formed tightly interlinked communities, known as bacterial colonies, and for billions of years, nature has maintained such communities at all levels of life. Natural selection favors those communities in which individuals act for the benefit of the community as a whole. In the human realm, we call this ethical behavior. So, ethics always has to do with community; it is behavior for the common good.

Today, we all belong to many communities, but we all share two communities to which we belong. We are all members of humanity, and we all belong to the global biosphere, the community of life. We are members of *oikos*, the Earth Household, which is the Greek root of "ecology." As members of the human community, our behavior should reflect a respect of human dignity and basic human rights.

As members of the Earth Household, we should behave as the other members of the household behave – the plants, animals, and microorganisms that form the vast network of relationships that we call the web of life. The outstanding characteristic of the biosphere is its inherent ability to sustain life. As members of the global community of living beings, it behooves us to behave in such a way that we respect, honor, and cooperate with nature's inherent ability to sustain life. As I have mentioned, this is the very essence of ecological sustainability.

Community and Transformative Learning

To summarize, meeting the challenge of ecological sustainability requires a profound change of concepts and ideas and also a profound change of values. This kind of learning is known as transformative learning. In my experience, the most powerful way to experience such transformative learning is through the experience of community. When you discuss systemic interconnectedness within a learning community, you experience human interconnectedness at the same time, and this is when transformative learning takes place most effectively. This is another reason why community is so important today.

Reference

Capra, F. and Luisi, P. L. (2014). *The systems view of life*. New York: Cambridge University Press.

VI

What Is Healing?

Chapter 16

What Is Called Healing?

M. Guy Thompson, PhD

What is healing? You would think that with all the attention we have paid to the notion of sanity and madness, health and sickness, well-being and misery throughout human history that we would have a fairly clear idea of what it means to be healthy. Sadly, this is not the case. As a topic in its own right it is seldom addressed, and when it is there is little insight into its nature. Even Buddhism, with its emphasis on achieving a more enlightened manner of living characterized by wisdom, rarely addresses the topic explicitly. Is the enlightened person healthier than the unenlightened, or is happiness a better determinant for a better life than enlightenment is? Wisdom and happiness are no doubt related. After all, Plato thought that wisdom was a *determinant* to happiness, though they are not interchangeable. Are we more sane the healthier we are, or is it possible to be sane and unhealthy? Or healthy and insane?

According to the Oxford English Dictionary, the word sane comes from the Latin *sanus*, meaning healthy or sound, as in sound mind and body. Herein lies the problem. If sanity means health, is it any wonder we are so muddled as to what it entails once we acknowledge we know just as little about health as we do about sanity? Medicine has traditionally defined health as the absence of disease or malady. This is the conceit of Western medicine, which endeavors to treat the illnesses it diagnoses with little awareness of the healthy condition it furthers. Unlike Chinese medicine, for example, which defines health as a state of wholeness and balance, Western medicine is content to treat illnesses by eradicating their toxic or otherwise unwelcome symptoms, hoping for the best outcome. If not a cure, then perhaps a reduction in suffering or prolongation of life, as in the old adage, "I dressed the wounds, but God cured him."

Western medicine has accomplished remarkable advances in the treatment of illness in spite of its narrow focus, but it also reminds us why Western medicine is ill-suited for "treating" what it portrays as a "mental illness." Psychiatry's strategy in treating mental states is virtually the same as when treating physical maladies: locate what is wrong and neutralize it. *Health*, whatever it is, will take care of itself. We are finally beginning to realize the limitations of Western medicine and focusing more deliberately on what health *is* and cultivating it thoughtfully. Isn't it about time we did the same for our minds?

DOI: 10.4324/9781003564294-22

What I want to explore in this essay is the nature of health, or healing, what it is, and how to effect it. In order to do this we will also touch on the notion of authenticity, a seminal concept in existential philosophy as well as in existential psychoanalysis. In order to get there, we will have to take a journey through the etymology of terms such as health and sanity to get to a notion of healing that we can relate to, and perhaps embrace. I hope in the end we will agree that health and authenticity are not only related but decisively so. But first, let us take a look at the word health and explore what this term can tell us.

Actually, the words health (or healthy) and sane (or sanity) are closely related. According to Partridge (1966), the word sane is cognate with the words sanitary, sanitation, and sanitarium, words with which we are all familiar. We usually think of sanitary as related to cleanliness, and it is, but only indirectly. Sanitary literally means healthy, but because a dirty kitchen or surgical theater is deemed unhealthy, the terms health and cleanliness became synonymous. On the other hand, a sanitarium is a place crazy people go to in order to become sane, as in "mental sanitarium" (as distinct from sanitariums that segregated persons suffering from tuberculosis before antibiotics were invented). Partridge tells us that the word sane is also akin to the Greek *iaino*, meaning "I heal," and cognate with the words health and healing. If sane or sanity means healthy or to heal, then what does health mean? Partridge tells us that the words heal and health come from the word "whole" (spelled with a W), which in turn is derived from the Middle English *hole* (spelled with an H) and Old English *hal*, meaning sound, as in sound body or mind, or the word "complete." You could say to be healthy is consistent with the feeling that there is nothing missing in your life. Does this mean that to be healthy or to heal means to make whole? The word whole gives rise to wholesome, which we typically associate with health. It also gives rise to the word hail, as in hailing a taxi. The origin of this expression, however, was used as a simple greeting, when shouting out "hail!" to an acquaintance, as in "be well." When we greet a friend with the salutation, "how are you?" we are inquiring into their health, which every one of us appears to be obsessed with. To "hail" also means to make well or to cure, so hail and heal are closely related, though not interchangeable.

To sum up, the word sane is cognate with the word health, which in turn goes back to the word whole, which, among other things, means sound or complete. Now we have to wonder, what does it mean to be sound? There are three meanings for the word sound; two are nouns which connote a body of water or a noise. The other is an adjective, and that is the one we want to look at. Partridge tells us that sound comes from the Old English *sund* and is akin to the Latin *sanus*, meaning flawless or unharmed. The Oxford English Dictionary expands on this further, suggesting that a sound person is free from disease, infirmity, or injury. It also means to be unimpaired, in good condition, wholesome, of solid or ample character, morally good, honest, sincere, and of sober or solid judgment (as in, one must be sober to judge effectively).

Now let us summarize what we have learned about the word sane and all its apparent permutations. Taken together via our etymological inventory, to be sane is to be healthy, to heal, to be whole, wholesome or complete, to be sound, to be well, and to make well or to cure. It also means to be flawless, unharmed, unimpaired, of solid character, morally good, honest, sincere, and of sober judgment. If all that is entailed in being sane, no wonder we seek it! It is worth noting at this juncture that the word wisdom, the objective of Buddhism, though not etymologically related, is nevertheless akin to sanity. The word wise derives from the word *vide*, which literally means to *see*. Derived from the Latin *uidere*, it is related to the Sanskrit words *veda* and *vedanta*, the Hindu word for knowledge. The word vide also gives us the words visa, envisage, visible, vision, visionary, visitor, advise, evidence, interview, improvise, review, revise, supervise, survey, clairvoyant, wit, wizard, and, of course, wise and wisdom. The Oxford English Dictionary defines wisdom as a manner, custom, and course of action, as in *likewise* and *otherwise*. The wise person possesses and exercises sound judgment and discernment, having the ability to perceive and adopt the best means to accomplish an end, qualities we attributed earlier to sanity.

As we now see, sanity and judgment are inextricably connected. But we have also seen that there is more to sanity than judgment alone. One of the most common ways of characterizing a crazy person is that he or she is "split" or broken. The schizophrenic suffers from a broken mind or heart. The paranoiac is literally "beside himself" (*para* = beside, *noos* = mind), split into two people or minds. Among psychoanalysts, splitting is embraced as the most prevalent symptom, or rather, defense mechanism of psychosis. If there is any truth to these assumptions, then it makes sense to think of health as the reverse of splitting, of becoming whole again, as in wholesome and solid, completely who you are. But health is more complicated than simply becoming a whole, solid person who had fallen apart, who had come apart at the seams and lost his or her bearings. It also implies the wherewithal of taking off the mask I was using to conceal myself from others, of coming out of the closet and becoming, perhaps for the first time, *who* I am, without fear of consequence. This is probably where the notion of honesty comes in and why that term is associated with becoming a sounder person. If pretending to be someone I am not is dishonest, then becoming who I am would entail honesty, to be genuine with myself and with others. When I am honest, I no longer need to effect the subterfuge that we associate with madness.

Now I want to turn our attention to the role that authenticity plays in health, which addresses the healing aspect of honesty. What does authenticity entail, and how does becoming more authentic heal and facilitate a more healthy and sane way of being with myself and with others? First I want to direct our attention to the work of D. W. Winnicott and review his conception of true and false-self phenomena. Winnicott never invoked the term authenticity specifically, but his conception of a true and false self enjoys important similarities. Moreover, Winnicott was one of R. D. Laing's supervisors when Laing was undergoing his psychoanalytic training at the British Psychoanalytic Society in the late 1950s during the period when both were developing their respective conceptions of the false-self system, Laing in *The Divided Self* (1960 [1969]) and Winnicott most notably in his (1960 [1976]) paper, "Ego Distortion in Terms of True and False-Self" published the same year Laing's book was published.

Winnicott believed that Freud's structural model of id, ego, and superego did not adequately address the problem of selfhood and that it was impossible to locate a personal self in Freud's schema. Was the ego the self, as Freud implied, or was the entire tripartite structure the self, but a divided one, which Freud also inferred? Winnicott introduced the notion of a *self*, borrowed from Jung, to connote both a personal and technical term that was more or less superimposed onto Freud's structural model, but intended to replace it. This decision was slightly problematic because Winnicott didn't really integrate his model with Freud's, but permitted them to exist side by side. Some have suggested this was a split in Winnicott's thinking. This was typical of Winnicott, a strategy he adopted when reconciling Melanie Klein's theories with his own – not entirely rejecting her theory but not integrating it with his either. Be that as it may, though Winnicott's theory of a false self lacks theoretical cohesion, it does compensate for the lack of a self in Freud's model.

Briefly, Winnicott posits a true self at the beginning of the child's development, while acknowledging that it shares similar qualities to Freud's conception of the id. Winnicott and Freud both believed that the child lacks an ego at this early stage and that the mother serves the function of an external ego for her baby, epitomized by Winnicott's unsettling statement that there is no such thing as "a baby" (without a mother to nurture it). The child begins to develop a "false" self after six months or so, as a normal part of its development, at exactly the same time that Freud believed that the ego begins to emerge from the id. Winnicott (1960 [1976], p. 140) admits that his conception of the true self shares similarities with the id, just as the false self shares similarities with the ego. However, at this juncture the similarities between Winnicott's and Freud's respective schemas ends. Though Winnicott held that the emergence of the false self is normative, he also believed that the baby may form its false self prematurely if the mother doesn't provide sufficient nurturing by intuitively understanding the baby's emotional needs. Should this happen (or, rather, not happen), the baby has no recourse but to reverse roles and undertake to "mother" its own mother (or primary caretaker) in order to secure its own welfare. This tactic, however, eventually results in negative and sometimes grave consequences.

Winnicott envisioned the true self as a term that connotes the totality of our emotions, where our sense of being originates. It is not literally a "self" in the sense of a *second* self to the one that is false. There is really only *one* self, but with private and public functions and qualities. Likewise, the so-called false self is not nearly as ominous as it sounds. A better term might have been the social self, because that is essentially what it is. As envisioned by Winnicott, the false self more or less exercises the synthetic functions of Freud's ego: negotiating social space, learning appropriate social cues in its conduct of interpersonal relationships, devising and executing courses of action, and developing ways of defending itself. We all need our false selves in order to deal with other people and compensate for our latent narcissism. It is the vehicle for our interpersonal relationships. However, if it takes over the function of navigating social space *before* the true self is able to flourish, the child may become compliant and eager to please at the expense of trusting other people. This person may alternately become downright hostile.

Though Winnicott and Laing each see the self as divided, they aren't suggesting there are literally *two* selves, one true and one false. In the healthy person, the true and false self aren't opposed but function in relative harmony. Those who engage in splitting harbor feelings so privately they have virtually lost touch with them. They're more devoted to procuring security than with securing love, though they often confuse the two. I may keep my feelings and desires not merely private but dark secrets I dare not confess or act upon.

Conclusion

In conclusion, equating heath and healing with making whole or complete would seem to be far more relevant to the manner with which a person conducts his or her life than with the navigation of physical illness or the incessant monitoring of pain and suffering. You might put it this way: that your life is empty, or barren, or that something is missing and you need to make it right. These manners of expression seem more relevant to life, love, and happiness – to *health* – than they do to treating COVID, or cancer, or a broken limb. In arriving at this conception of health, perhaps the Greeks believed that health relies on a healthy and vibrant *life*. The problem with the medical model is that it is rooted in the body and the relative absence of pain or infirmity, which is an inadequate foundation for living a happy – which is to say *healthy* – life. Any psychiatry, for example, that administers medication exclusively relies on suppressing or tranquilizing painful feelings instead of locating such feelings in the manner by which we conduct our lives. Talking therapy isn't intended to suppress our experiences or hide from our problems, but to explore, understand, and come to terms with them, without fear or resentment.

This, it seems to me, is what being healthy is essentially about.

References

Laing, R. D. (1960[1969]). *The divided self.* New York and London: Penguin Books.

Partridge, E. (1966). *Origins: A short etymological dictionary of modern English,* 4th ed. London: Routledge and Kegan Paul.

Winnicott, D. W. (1960[1976]). Ego distortion in terms of true and false self. In *The maturational processes and the facilitating environment: Studies in the theory of emotional development.* London: The Hogarth Press.

Chapter 17

Healing and the Regeneration of Life

Fritjof Capra, PhD

I would like to begin with the observation that it is impossible to give a precise definition of health. Health is to a large extent a subjective experience whose quality can be known intuitively but can never be exhaustively described or quantified. What we can say is that health is a state of well-being that arises when the organism functions in a certain way.

The description of this way of functioning will depend on how we describe the organism. This means that our understanding of health will always be linked to our understanding of life. Different models of living organisms will lead to different definitions of health.

I have spent the last few decades developing a synthesis of a new understanding of life which has emerged at the forefront of science (see Capra and Luisi, 2014). I call my synthesis "the systems view of life" because it involves systemic thinking, or "systems thinking" – thinking in terms of relationships, patterns, and context.

I would like to briefly summarize this systems view of life and then propose a corresponding systems view of health and healing.

The Systems View of Life

According to the systems view, the central characteristic of biological life is what poets and sages throughout the ages have called "the breath of life." In modern scientific language, it is known as metabolism, defined as a ceaseless flow of energy and matter through a network of chemical processes, which enables a living organism to continually regenerate itself. As the great microbiologist Lynn Margulis (1999) used to say: "If it metabolizes, it's alive; if it doesn't metabolize, it is not alive."

The understanding of metabolism includes two basic aspects: flows and networks. Let me begin with networks. The network is the basic pattern of organization of all living systems. Ecosystems are networks of organisms, organisms are networks of tissues and cells, cells are networks of molecules, and social systems are networks of communications. Wherever we see life, we see networks.

The key characteristic of these living networks is that they are self-generating; they continually regenerate themselves by transforming or replacing their

DOI: 10.4324/9781003564294-23

components (see Capra, 2024). Now the continual regeneration of life in nature is ancient knowledge. You just have to look at the turning of the seasons and new growth in spring. What is new in the systems view is that this regeneration operates at all levels of life, down to the molecular networks in cells.

Regeneration is the very essence of the life process. When regeneration stops, life stops. In a more philosophical vein, we might even say that regeneration is the purpose of life or the meaning of life.

The continual regeneration of living networks, of transforming and replacing their components, requires continual flows of energy and matter. This is how the network aspect of metabolism is linked to the flow aspect.

The next important observation is that as these metabolic flows go through networks, they will include cyclical pathways. So, now we have networks, flows, and cycles as key concepts. These cycles can act as feedback loops, which allow the living network to regulate itself and to organize itself. Feedback may either be self-balancing or self-amplifying. Self-amplifying, or "runaway," feedback may lead to points of instability where there is either a breakdown or a spontaneous emergence of new order.

This spontaneous emergence of new order at critical points of instability, often referred to just as "emergence," implies that creativity – the generation of new forms – is a key property of all living systems. Life is inherently creative.

And finally, I want to mention the special way in which living systems interact with their environment. A living organism responds to influences from its environment with structural changes, and it does so autonomously, specifying which influences to notice and how to respond according to its nature and previous experience. This type of response is defined as cognitive. Continual cognitive interactions with the environment are an essential part of an organism's metabolism, and thus life and cognition are inseparably linked: life is inherently intelligent.

The Systems View of Health

Let me now outline a systems view of health corresponding to the systems view of life. The systems view sees life as organizing itself in networks that are inherently regenerative, sustained by continual flows of energy and matter. In other words, life is a process, or a network of processes. Therefore, health, too, must be understood as a process rather than a static state of perfect well-being.

Moreover, the systems view integrates several dimensions of life. Accordingly, the process of health is also seen as multidimensional with mutually interacting biological, cognitive, social, and environmental dimensions.

To get a more detailed idea of the process of health, we can start from the observation that all living networks have feedback loops embedded in them, as I have mentioned. This results in a stability that is totally dynamic, characterized by continual interdependent fluctuations. The more dynamic the state of the system, the greater its flexibility, its ability to adapt to environmental changes. Loss of flexibility means loss of health.

Based on this view of living systems, I have proposed a systemic definition of health as "a state of well-being, resulting from a dynamic balance that involves the physical and psychological aspects of the organism, as well as its interactions with its natural and social environment" (Capra, 1982, p. 323).

This definition of health allows us to understand the potential of self-healing inherent in every living organism. It is the organism's innate tendency to regenerate itself in a balanced state when it has been disturbed. In other words, health and healing are seen as particular processes of regeneration. Healing may involve returning to a previous balanced state, or it may involve stages of crisis and transformation – the manifestations of life's creativity – resulting in an entirely new balanced state.

I want to mention that, to my knowledge, the first to see healing as a process of crisis and transformation, as breakthrough rather than breakdown, was R. D. Laing (1967) several decades before this process, now known as emergence, was discovered and explored in the language of complexity theory.

Finally, we need to remember that, according to the systems view, life is inherently intelligent, because the interactions of a living organism with its environment are cognitive interactions. This includes in particular the processes of getting sick and of healing. In other words, there is a cognitive, or mental, dimension in every illness, even if it often lies in the realm of the unconscious.

References

Capra, F. (1982). *The turning point*. New York: Simon and Schuster.
Capra, F. (2024). *Systemic principles of life*. Resurgence (UK), to be published.
Capra, F. and Luisi, P. L. (2014). *The systems view of life*. New York: Cambridge University Press.
Laing, R. D. (1967). *The politics of experience*. New York: Ballantine.
Margulis, L. (1999). Personal communication.

Chapter 18

Laing and the Human Condition

Douglas Kirsner, PhD

Ever since my undergraduate days in the 1960s, I have been taken with R. D. Laing. During 1975 and 1976 I had the good fortune of spending some months living in 74 Portland Road in London, the Philadelphia Association (PA) household that Hugh Crawford ran (to the extent that anyone could run it!). That is where Mike Thompson and I met, and we have remained close friends for the next half century!

In the basement of that house was the headquarters of the PA, which R. D. Laing still actively chaired. (Only "chaired" since it was next to impossible to lead such an eccentric bunch of individualistic sceptics; in any case, Laing seemed constitutionally unable to keep many followers for long.) Down there it was like the Freudian unconscious – anarchic, timeless, creative, unconventional and unpredictable though to some extent interpretable. It was really an anti-organization where rules were left at the top of the stairs. As home to the PA's many seminars and workshops, there was always some activity, at least from late afternoon on. When there weren't animated seminars (dwelling, existentialism, psychoanalysis, phenomenology, asylums, etc.), yoga and meditation workshops were taking place.

Down there, on the side, was Mike Thompson's office. He was then secretary of the PA. Bob Dylan had just released his album *Desire*, and Mike played it all the time for months on end. We always had one more cup of coffee for the road!

I was beguiled. I had been interested in Laing for years and even written a book, *The Schizoid World of Jean-Paul Sartre and R. D. Laing* (Kirsner, 1976 [2003]). I argued there that both Sartre and his disciple Laing started out from a schizoid problematic, one which nonetheless addressed very real and significant psychosocial problems in the modern world. So in the Portland Road basement by day, I found myself rummaging through some of the old PA archives, reading Laing's careful notes of Sartre's works. At night, I attended lectures and seminars, including Laing's ruminative lectures, which were at that time certainly quite wonderfully absorbing and creative.

Of course, I spent time with Laing and other members of the PA. I once asked Laing why his general influence was not that great. He replied that there was no Laingian technique, there was no Laingian School. I am sure he was right – although there was no particular healing technique, there was a philosophy.

DOI: 10.4324/9781003564294-24

But there was more. Although he was charismatic, Laing's personality was such that he could not really sustain a movement with disciples. He was often narcissistic and could appear as a trickster, somebody indefinable and unpredictable. A skeptic at heart, he was no dogmatist. He was a chameleon who was not graspable in his essence. People had very different takes on who their "Ronnie" was and what he allegedly believed in. Nobody owned him, not the left, the anti-psychiatrists, the Buddhists, not even the PA that he founded.

It's hard these days to conceptualize how really famous Laing was in his heyday. A wide range of groups wanted to claim him for their own – from young to old, from left to right, from yin to yang. But factors including the Vietnam War, the May 68 revolution, the counterculture, the pill, the time of sex and drugs and psychedelic music combined to make the zeitgeist for Laing to make a huge impact. Although he obviously loved being so famous, Laing could not relish it properly since he was always frightened of losing his identity by being categorized. Laing was star-struck by his own image, overawed by his own reputation and role. This was strange for such a serious student of Sartre on self-deception – he seemed to have the delusion that he was "R. D. Laing".

In any case, fortunately, Laing was never reducible to his reputation. When Sartre was asked why he was studying Paul Valéry who his critics dismissed as merely a "bourgeois intellectual", Sartre responded that while it was certainly true that Valéry was a bourgeois intellectual, not every bourgeois intellectual was Paul Valéry. I felt the same about Laing. While Laing no doubt had major problems (alcohol, drugs, narcissism, etc.), there can be no doubt that, despite these problems, he made exceptional contributions.

What were these exceptional contributions? I think his major contributions to healing lay in some of his own qualities, his general sensibility, approach and philosophy – perhaps apparently simple things like listening, respect, staying and sticking with the person, allowing them to "be" themselves and then move on from there in understanding what is going on in some form or other. That isn't the same as agreeing with the patient, but of healing as holistic, the whole picture of a person. Beyond Laing's personal qualities that lay the ground, it was his focus on communications, psychological contexts of social groupings and their histories that the person is involved with. In fact, I think what has been often missed is that whatever else he was involved in thinking about, Laing was at bottom focused throughout his work on communication – how we do or don't communicate, levels and meta-levels of communication and mystification, and situation within context.

Throughout his varied career Laing focused on many things: schizophrenia, birth and pre-birth experience, the family, the impact of the modern world of science and technology, yoga, politics, the impact of psychiatry, patients' rights, the vagaries of love and many more. But there was a vital link permeating all of them which originated with what is central to Sartre – the distinction between two realms, *the human and the nonhuman and the consequences of treating human beings as though they were objects or things*. Like Sartre, who began with the radical ontological division of the world into human and nonhuman, "being for-itself" and "being-in-itself", existence and essence, free and unfree, Laing took as his starting point that no matter how alienated, every human being was free and needed to be treated as a free agent who could not avoid making choices. On this premise, it is inappropriate to talk about human beings in "thing" language; language about things or processes is never appropriate for ultimately understanding human beings.

While Laing was influenced by many philosophers and psychoanalysts, the extent to which Laing followed Sartre's philosophy has been underrated. In fact, I do not believe that Laing can be fully appreciated without recognizing the central role of Sartre's philosophy his own work, for their starting points which divided being itself into free and determined beings were identical. Without recognizing Laing's allegiance to Sartre's standpoint, many of Laing's interests and perspectives appear unconnected and arbitrary. Laing's fascination with Sartre went back to his youth. David Cooper told me how Laing pored over Sartre's *Being and Nothingness* through many nights, black coffee at his side. Laing and Cooper published their summaries of some of Sartre's later work, including his *Critique of Dialectical Reason* to which Sartre wrote an appreciative foreword in 1963. It is worth quoting from it:

> Like you I think that we cannot understand psychic troubles *from outside* . . . I believe also that one cannot study nor cure a neurosis without an original respect for the person of the patient . . . I maintain like you I believe, mental illness to be the issue that the free organism, in its total unity, invents to live in an unliveable situation. For that reason, I attach the greatest value to your research, in particular to the study that you have made of the family milieu taken as group and as series and I am convinced that your efforts contribute to our approaching the time when psychiatry will be, finally, *human*.
>
> (Sartre, *Foreword*, Laing and Cooper, 1964, my translation)

"Finally human" – quite a statement of values. Clearly, Sartre assumed that mainstream psychiatry treated people as things. Sartre took it as axiomatic that the human world was based on our praxis, agency and freedom and was irreducible to definitions of essences. Our being was always in question. Laing's landscape was essentially Sartre's – our essential freedom, self-deception, experience and its violation, the terror of the group, fear and intrusion of others, mystification, being for others as hostility and objectification. First and foremost, we must understand human beings as agents, as producers, as praxis. For Sartre, our behavior was always intelligible, and it was self-deception to ignore that. Since we started as agents who were condemned to be free, we could not escape our freedom. On the other hand, the nonhuman world was that of things, of identities, of essences and processes.

Laing took the implications of Sartre's schema very seriously, which has important implications about healing. A "science of persons" and not of things was central to *The Divided Self* (Laing, 1965). Laing's abiding concern was with the implications of the intrusion of natural science into the human arena such as the scientific look or birth as an exclusively medical rather than a human event. For the schizophrenics of *The Divided Self*, the fact that they were persons meant that they were free and (if they wanted) could produce potentially intelligible communications through their actions. Word salads were red herrings produced to mystify others (they may also have helped to mystify themselves). Laing claimed that the schizophrenics deemed by conventional psychiatry to be beyond all reason as victims of illness processes could be regarded instead as agents whose experience was potentially understandable and rational when seen as intentional acts within a context. They were using Sartrean self-deception as a way of trying to live in what they saw to be an unlivable situation. But why would one not want to be free? For Sartre, the answer was clear: with freedom comes responsibility which cannot be avoided. Laing almost certainly overrated the magnitude of the patient's choices in schizophrenia – by challenging the role of unconscious factors as well as organic ones, he was left with little alternative. But he had tried to redress the balance a little in favor of the schizophrenic as human and acting meaningfully rather than as merely the victim of an organic process. The idea of treating a patient with respect and of listening and recognition as agents may not be sufficient for healing but is in truth at least necessary to get onto the road to recovery.

For Sartre whose collected essays appeared as a series entitled *Situations*, all free human actions took place within a setting, within certain parameters, as though they were on a stage where although the scene was set, the actors could script the actions. For Sartre, all actions occurred within a structured context which impacted in a specific way with a particular person. Like Sartre, Laing always focused on *context* as a way of understanding those social events which seemed irrational. If we situate the context, we may better empathize with the specific intentions of the free subject. Laing utilized a systems theory approach with the concept of meta-context – the context of a context – to understand the hidden rationality in a situation, especially because meta-contexts by definition were not observable.

Laing completed *The Divided Self* in 1956 before Sartre published *Search for a Method* and *Critique of Dialectical Reason* in 1960. After *The Divided Self* Laing moved from an interest in the meaning in the intrapsychic life of the individual through the context of interpersonal space of two persons (*Self and Others*) which, following the later Sartre, is locatable within the group or family context. In *Sanity, Madness and the Family* (with Esterson) and *The Politics of the Family* Laing was interested in how the family constellation provided the context in which individual schizophrenic experience could be understood as a rational strategy. For Sartre and Laing, this group context existed within a society which was part of the context of the total social world system, which is in turn part of the cosmos. In *The Politics of Experience* Laing understood the total social world system as providing the social context in which schizophrenia was an understandable reaction. In *Knots* and also in parts of *The Politics of Experience* Laing even allowed for the possibility of mystical experience to explain seemingly irrational experience and behavior in terms of the biggest meta-context of all. Mysticism was about as far as contextualizing could go, and Laing went to Ceylon to meditate in 1971.

Of course, Sartre was too much of a rationalist to make Laing's further move of situating the social world within the mystical. But the methodology of investigating specific "situations" illuminates Laing's basic approach and abiding project because, like Sartre, Laing appreciated individuals in their singularity at the same time as they represented something more general. *Context* for Sartre and Laing was the human equivalent to cause in the nonhuman world. To the extent that context provided the parameters of choice, we are all, in Sartre's term, "universal singulars" where we can cross-reference an individual with his or her time. Laing was sensitive to and respected the unique experience of individuals whom he did not suppose that he understood because he was an "expert" in mental illness. When he wanted, Laing had an uncanny ability to hear and empathize. Empathy, respect and listening are helpful for Laing's contribution to healing, but additionally an *understanding context* is vital.

Laing was to psychotics what Freud was to neurotics – he listened to their stories to help understand their meaning in terms of wishes and intentions, not of organic processes. Challenging conventional mores and approaches, Laing was, as Mike Thompson has pointed out, in the Greek tradition of skepticism where little or nothing was taken for granted. Dichotomies, such as "inside-outside", "mind-body", "self-other", "society-individual", "mad-normal" were, as he would have put it, "up for grabs". Philosophy, especially existential philosophy and phenomenology, suffused his work with the clinical data gleaned from his work as a psychiatrist and psychoanalyst as live material to further explore the humanity or lack of it in the human world. Laing was particularly offended by the stand of Karl Jaspers and modern psychiatry that there was a category of human beings – psychotics – who were "un-understandable". There was, according to Jaspers, an unbridgeable "abyss of difference" between psychotics and the rest of us (Kirsner, 1990). Not that there weren't some obvious differences, but they were, for Laing, a challenge rather than a bridge that could never be crossed. For Laing, whatever else it was, schizophrenia was always a social event taking place within a social context needing to be understood to situate the experience and behavior of the psychotic. Whatever might be happening inside the person, clearly there were dramatic and significant events occurring outside, in interpersonal space and outside that in the broader social contexts. Laing was the major figure who helped loosen up the mind-set of "us" the normal versus "them" the mad. He was bent on searching for the interpersonal and social context of the diagnosis of psychosis and its impact.

Moreover, there was the issue of perspective – radically different consequences accrue from the initial stance of seeing someone as a person or as an object. Since the observer was always part of the observational field, how one treated someone impacted how they reacted and how they were seen. Along with phenomenological thinkers in general, for Sartre, consciousness was never independent but always consciousness of something – one's stance determined what one saw. This phenomenology of ways of seeing is clear in Laing from the beginning. In *The Divided Self* Laing wrote:

> Man's being . . . can be seen from different points of view and one or other aspect can be made the focus of study. In particular, man can be seen as a person or thing. Now, even the same thing, seen from different points of view, gives rise to two entirely different descriptions, and the descriptions give rise to two entirely different theories, and the theories result in two entirely different sets of action. The initial way we see a thing gives rise to all our subsequent dealings with it.

> (1965, p. 20)

Laing took the implications of one's point of view much further in his later work – he made the concept of "the normal" itself a focus of investigation and critique. This is epitomized in one of Laing's very best pieces, "The Obvious", Laing's contribution to the Dialectics of Liberation conference in 1967 (Laing, 1968).

Etymologically, the "obvious" is that which stands in front of us. The story Laing told about the woman holding her three-year-old out of a sixth-story window to show how much she loved him by not dropping him was, for Laing, an example of the crazed terrorism of hyper-normality. The normal stance for Laing was so warped as to be anti-human, as not treating people with the respect and dignity appropriate to human beings. Our reflex to obey, encapsulated in the Milgram experiments, was the result of treating people as though they were behaviorist machines. The double meaning of "diagnosis" as "*seeing* through" or seeing *through* social reality demonstrated the central issue that the perspective one adopted determined what one saw. Treating humans as persons had vastly different consequences from treating them as machines or things.

In Laing's later work the basically subjective and human was made to stand in stark contrast to a technocratic and objective scientific approach. Thus, his interest in the birth process, pre-birth experience, the way the mind has been seen in mechanistic terms and the technological worldview of knowledge without love can be seen in the context of Laing's interest in human agency as a primary explanatory factor in the human world. After *Knots* (1970), he wrote a play, *Do You Love Me?* (1972), a self-indulgent book of Laing's conversations with his children and another self-indulgent book, this time of sonnets. However, there was also *The Facts of Life* (1976), where he investigated the possibility of pre-birth experience as providing a template for later seemingly unintelligible behavior and experience. He raised the question as to what would happen to our worldview if we allowed ourselves to think whether there was some degree of intentionality in life before birth. It also focused on pre-birth experience and the technological fix of psychiatry. *The Voice of Experience* (1982) discussed experience, technology, psychiatry and once again the possibility of pre-birth experience, and *Wisdom, Madness and Folly* (1985) was an autobiography of his early years and his years of becoming a psychiatrist.

Freud thought that slips of the tongue and other marginalia of the psychopathology of everyday life could provide us with important discoveries about the nature of the human mind. I think that for Laing schizophrenia played a similar role in providing a way into understanding the lost world of human experiencing. I think one of the reasons that Laing so often felt he had been misunderstood is that his project was far larger than understanding schizophrenia. It is as though Freud were saddled with the discovery of Freudian slips as his major achievement – Freudian slips were a waystation and not any kind of endpoint. I think Laing's endpoint is the role of the loss of the world of valid experience as the problem of our age. This has consequences for our view of the world beyond "normality", such as the place of science and how alienated medicine becomes when we think that it is an achievement for a woman to be able to read a newspaper while she is having a baby. Issues about the central denial and violation of the realm of experience in the modern world persisted for Laing until the end of his life. They are evidenced by Laing's interest in Francis Mott's strange ideas about pre-birth experience, the importance of the voice of experience and its relation to the scientific "look", the asylum post–Kingsley Hall communities in London which were all aspects of a living phenomenology, what we did to ourselves and others in order to not see what we experience. Scientific objective rationality systematically contributed to the destruction and invalidation of the primacy of experience as providing specifically human data. In his social phenomenology Laing illuminated a specific type of *sensibility* to experience, a natural way of being alive to oneself and others which he felt had been lost.

Of course, there was his last yet unpublished book about love, an issue which pervades his work. How is love between two human beings possible? If we love somebody, we love them as they are in their own being, or "is-ness". To love somebody, for Laing, is to leave them alone as they are in their unique difference from us. For Laing, the modern world seemed beholden to a soulless scientific "knowledge without love", as the astronomer, C. F. von Weizsacker put it (see Laing, 1976, p. 142). How could a knowledge without love yield a knowledge of love? From Laing's perspective, the only way to humanize science was for it to assume human premises.

How was love possible in the modern world in which people seemed increasingly to be treated as objects? The name of the organization he founded with others in 1964 to deal with human distress, the Philadelphia Association (PA), was derived from the idea of "brotherly love". The PA's main concern was with people "whose relations with themselves and others have become an occasion of wretchedness" and to "come to a better understanding of how we occasion our suffering and joy, of the ways we may lose ourselves and each other, and find ourselves and each other again". Laing was always concerned with the disjunctions between people which prevented simple, natural love from occurring. For Sartre and Laing, no matter how alienated we humans are from ourselves or others, we are always free agents to some extent. The assumptions of science where it involved humans demanded fundamental questioning for Laing since the starting points of the human and nonhuman approaches were radically different and thus led to different conclusions. Treating persons as things implied that one inevitably reached conclusions about things and not people. That was Laing's basic existential critique of psychiatry, which was a paradigmatic instance of a "heartless" approach that no matter how "humane" was fundamentally flawed by confusing people with things, talking about humans in nonhuman terms. That is why "experience" is such a basic datum for Laing and the violation and mystification of experience was always so important and why "sensibility" to the nuances of others' experience was so essential for Laing. Therefore, the underlying reason that Laing focused so much on "the scientific look", on the heartlessness of psychiatry, on invalidation and the circles of deceit which lead to mystification and on the difficulties of love (of oneself and others) was the degree to which (even inadvertently) we treat others or ourselves as things instead of as free agents. Laing argued from *The Divided Self* onward that there was a world of difference between treating somebody as a victim of processes or as a being whose actions were the result of intentions.

Laing's approach was existential, phenomenological and experiential – concepts such as "ontological insecurity", invalidation and mystification of experience, alienation from who we and others are and the impact of deception were definitively human terms for understanding the human situation. In one lecture I recall, mentioned in Chapter 12, Laing telling of the impact on an elderly woman when she found out that her husband had been having an affair for 40 years. Her whole sense of reality was destroyed. The problem was not so much the affair as the effect on her sense of who she was having lived with such a fundamental deception for so long. What perception or what person could now be worthy of trust?

In his 1964 Preface to the Pelican Edition of *The Divided Self*, Laing wrote:

> Freud insisted that our civilization is a repressive one. There is a conflict between the demands of conformity and the demands of our instinctive energies, explicitly sexual. Freud could see no easy resolution of this antagonism, and he came to believe that in our time the possibility of simple natural love between human beings had already been abolished.
>
> (Laing, 1965, p. 11)

During my 1980 interview about the human condition, Laing reminded me again of Freud's comment I referred to in Chapter 12. This is the passage from *Civilization and Its Discontents*:

> Among the works of the sensitive English writer, John Galsworthy . . . there is a short story of which I early formed a high opinion. It is called "The Apple-Tree", and it brings home to us how the life of present-day civilized people leaves no room for the simple natural love of two human beings.
>
> (Freud, 1930, p. 105)

I think that this passage indicates something central to Laing's own abiding view of the world so vividly expressed in *The Politics of Experience*, Laing's version of *Civilization and Its Discontents*. It is scarcely accidental that Laing's last and unfinished work was devoted to the history of love. But while the regrets for what has been lost may be similar for Freud and Laing, Laing's view strongly contrasts to Freud's. Laing was an irremediable romantic, reminiscent of Jean-Jacques Rousseau who argued for the natural goodness of men and women before their corruption by civilization: "Man is born free but everywhere he is in chains". We cannot predict, Laing once said, the behavior of animals in their natural state from the behavior of animals in captivity. Freud adopted a tragic view of human existence which assumed malaise to be inherent in culture – Freud, like Sartre, held an anti-romantic Hobbesian view of the human condition. Laing diverged greatly from Sartre on this issue. For Sartre, the problems of human relationships were not attributable to human history, but were inscribed in the nature of being-for-others itself. But for Laing, our problems lie ultimately in treating people as objects and not as human. I think Laing's view of human nature, certainly as expressed in *The Politics of Experience*, was a romantic one: we are inherently and naturally good if only the world would leave us alone. Love was possible if not for the inroads of civilization. Schizophrenics might be in a better state if only psychiatrists would not interfere with them. And people would be more human if technocrats did not treat them as things. We get the sense of a simple, natural human situation from which we have become estranged. On this view, we are, as the Scottish Christians of his youth would have put it, "corrupted".

Perhaps Laing romanticized what it is to be human partly in reaction to the prevalent ways of looking at humans in nonhuman terms. But his strength lay in his stance as a skeptic who challenged the presumption of knowledge by those who looked at humans from a standpoint appropriate for looking at things. Some of his popularity was in his questioning of established claims to knowledge, especially around mental illness issues. His strength lay in his questioning the impact of looking at the human world in nonhuman terms and in providing glimpses of the possibilities of a more human world where relationships were a good deal more humane.

Nobody could deny that Laing, in the words of one of his favorite philosophers, Friedrich Nietzsche, would always "live dangerously".

For me the vagaries, complexities, strengths and weaknesses of Laing's life and work can be summed up in another of Nietzsche's memorable phrases – Ronnie Laing was "human, all too human".

References

Freud, S. (1930). Civilization and its discontents. In *The standard edition of the complete psychological works of Sigmund Freud*, Vol. XXI, pp. 57–146 (1927–1931): The Future of an Illusion, Civilization and its discontents, and other works. London: Hogarth Press and the Institute of Psychoanalysis.

Kirsner, D. (1976[2003]). *The schizoid world of Jean-Paul Sartre and R. D. Laing*. Hillsdale, NJ: Humanities Press/Brisbane: University of Queensland Press/New York: Other Press.

Kirsner, D. (1990). Across an abyss: Laing, Jaspers and Sartre. *Journal of the British Society for Phenomenology*, 21, no. 3: 209–216.

Laing, R. D. (1965). *The divided self.* New York: Pelican.

Laing, R. D. (1968). The obvious. In D. Cooper (ed.), *The dialectics of liberation*, pp. 13–33. Harmondsworth: Penguin Books.

Laing, R. D. (1970). *Knots.* London: Tavistock.

Laing, R. D. (1972). *Do you love me? An entertainment in conversation and verse.* New York: Pantheon.

Laing, R. D. (1976). *The facts of life.* London: Allen Lane.

Laing, R. D. (1982). *The voice of experience.* London: Allen Lane.

Laing, R. D. (1985). *Wisdom, madness and folly: The making of a psychiatrist.* London: Macmillan.

Laing, R. D. and Cooper, D. G. (1964). *Reason and violence: A decade of Sartre's philosophy (1950–1960).* London: Tavistock.

Index

For Product Safety Concerns and Information please contact our EU
representative GPSR@taylorandfrancis.com
Taylor & Francis Verlag GmbH, Kaufingerstraße 24, 80331 München, Germany

www.ingramcontent.com/pod-product-compliance
Lightning Source LLC
Chambersburg PA
CBHW070711280326
41926CB00089B/3899